'This book is essential for all practitioners who use complementary therapies in their practice, or advise pregnant women about the use of complementary therapies. The book focusses on the fundamentals of safe and effective practice; challenging the misconception that the use of complementary therapies is safe for all women. Excellent evidenced-based reading. Highly recommended.'

– Louise Simpson, Consultant Midwife who utilises complementary therapies in her everyday practice to maximise normality in childbirth

'Anyone involved in complementary therapies and maternity will treasure this book. It provides teachings from a bio-psycho-social approach based on evidence-based practice. It demonstrates Denise's experience, passion and drive to educate professionals about complementary therapies while highlighting safety and professional accountability when using complementary therapies in maternity care.'

– Amanda Redford, Senior Research Midwife/Trial Co-ordinator, Acupuncturist and Complementary Healthcare Practitioner for Women's Health

of related interest

Essential Oils
A Handbook for Aromatherapy Practice Second Edition
Jennifer Peace Rhind
ISBN 978 1 84819 089 4
eISBN 978 0 85701 072 8

Aromatherapy vs MRSA
Antimicrobial Essential Oils to Combat Bacterial Infection,
Including the Superbug
Maggie Tisserand
ISBN 978 1 84819 237 9
eISBN 978 0 85701 191 6

Aromatica
A Clinical Guide to Essential Oil Therapeutics
Volume 1: Principles and Profiles
Peter Holmes LAc, MH
ISBN 978 1 84819 303 1
eISBN 978 0 85701 257 9

Aromatherapy in Midwifery Practice

Denise Tiran

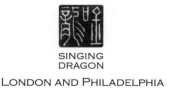

SINGING
DRAGON
LONDON AND PHILADELPHIA

First published in 2016
by Singing Dragon
an imprint of Jessica Kingsley Publishers
73 Collier Street
London N1 9BE, UK
and
400 Market Street, Suite 400
Philadelphia, PA 19106, USA

www.singingdragon.com

Library of Congress Cataloging in Publication Data
A CIP catalog record for this book is available from the Library of Congress

British Library Cataloguing in Publication Data
A CIP catalogue record for this book is available from the British Library

ISBN 978 1 84819 288 1
eISBN 978 0 85701 235 7

Printed and bound in Great Britain

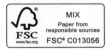

For Adam, with all my love

Acknowledgements

I would like to thank my editor, Claire Wilson, for giving me the opportunity to write this new textbook on aromatherapy in midwifery. I have known Claire for many years, since the first two editions of my previous book on the subject were published. It is exciting to be working with Claire again and in a new company, at a time when aromatherapy has become almost a standard part of pregnancy for many women.

I would particularly like to thank my partner, Dr Harry Chummun, lecturer in physiology at the University of Greenwich in London, the Open University and Expectancy (my company, which provides complementary therapy courses for midwives). His help in reading Chapter 3 on the science of aromatherapy has been invaluable and his support at home has allowed me time to work on the manuscript.

Thanks also go to my colleagues, Charlotte Kenyon, Deputy Head of Education at Expectancy and midwifery lecturer at the University of Huddersfield, as well as Expectancy's Programmes Administrator, Anoushka Lucas Howells. They have both taken off some of the pressure whilst I was completing the manuscript and have been a huge moral support to me. Charlotte in particular has been a source of help when I have needed to 'off-load' or to debate professional issues, either in relation to the content of the book, or in my ongoing teaching.

A huge thank you, too, to all the midwives who have attended Expectancy courses on aromatherapy and whose questions and discussions have highlighted the issues which midwives need to know in relation to using aromatherapy in their practice, particularly in the National Health Service.

Most of all, as ever, my love and gratitude go to my wonderful son, Adam. I first started writing books when he was only three years old so he has been with me throughout all the trials and tribulations which come with writing a book. At one time, Adam helped with some of the work in Expectancy, but he is now settled in London and working in the African music business. He is my most ardent supporter and I could not have done it without him in my life.

Denise Tiran MSc RM PGCEA

Contents

List of Boxes, Tables and Figures

Boxes

Tables

Figures

Introduction

I have been working in the specialist field of midwifery complementary medicine for over 30 years and have previously written several books for midwives on different aspects of this vast subject. My first book, *Complementary Therapies in Pregnancy and Childbirth*, was published in 1994 at a time when complementary therapies were still seen as rather strange alternative practices which did not fit well with conventional healthcare. Two editions of *Aromatherapy in Pregnancy and Childbirth* were published – in 1999 and 2004 – at a time when the general public, not least midwives and pregnant women, were becoming increasingly interested in using natural remedies.

In the 1980s and 1990s, I worked at what eventually became the University of Greenwich in southeast London as a midwifery lecturer. Given my area of expertise, I was fortunate to be given the opportunity to develop and manage first a Diploma of Higher Education and then a Bachelor of Science honours degree in complementary therapies, within which we included a pathway on aromatherapy. I also ran a specialist complementary therapy clinic at one of the local maternity units where student midwives undertook their clinical practice. I was able to use this as a teaching clinic for the student midwives and for students on the degree programme so that they could see complementary therapies in practice specifically applied to maternity care.

Over the next decade I treated almost 6000 pregnant and labouring women with complementary therapies, primarily aromatherapy, reflex zone therapy (a form of reflexology), massage, moxibustion for breech presentation and several other therapies. We had many visitors to the clinic, from both the United Kingdom and overseas, and were 'highly commended' in the 2001 Prince of Wales' Awards for Healthcare in London, as an example of the integration of complementary therapies within conventional healthcare.

By 2004 I had realised that 'complementary therapies' was a subject which was here to stay and that maternity care was one of the clinical fields in which it had become popular (oncology and palliative care were the only clinical fields in which complementary medicine was used more than in midwifery).

I had also recognised that midwives and some obstetricians wanted to access high-calibre training courses on a range of complementary therapies so that they could apply it to their practice, even if that was only to be able to give advice to women. At the same time, practitioners working in complementary therapies were beginning to look beyond generic practice merely as an aid to stress relief and relaxation and wanted to specialise in specific clinical fields. Maternity care was one of the most popular areas, but practitioners did not know where to find suitable training courses.

As a result, I took the huge, rather scary step to leave the university sector and to establish my own company. Expectancy (www.expectancy.co.uk) was born in 2004 and is now nearly 12 years down the line. Expectancy is an education company providing complementary therapy study days, short courses and long programmes of study for midwives, doulas, maternity support workers, maternity nurses, antenatal teachers and complementary therapists wanting to specialise in maternity work. We have an annual series of scheduled courses in the London area as well as providing in-house courses for maternity units and universities in the United Kingdom and overseas.

Self-employment in the commercial sector has brought with it many difficulties, not least in terms of learning how to run a business, market it, deal with the competition, cope with financial and legal requirements and so much more. It has also presented me with a significant conflict in terms of being an academic and a clinician versus the need to maintain the commercial side of the business. At heart I am a midwife and always will be. I am also a teacher and gain great satisfaction from enthusing others to take up the baton and to learn how to use complementary therapies for the benefit of mothers and babies. I also regard myself as a scientist, basing my teaching on the bio-psycho-social approach and ensuring that what I teach is based on contemporary evidence. Unfortunately, these high principles do not always go well with the commercial focus of making money and I have steadfastly refused to compromise my integrity by 'dumbing down' in order to attract more business. My personal philosophy of safety, professional accountability and evidence-based practice has become the company's philosophy and underpins all our educational activities and products. I have built my reputation on this philosophy and guard it jealously from any attempts to trivialise the subject matter, which can be very difficult on occasions.

Over the last 12 years I have worked with over 2000 midwives wanting to implement complementary therapies such as aromatherapy in their practice, as well as numerous therapists wishing to work with pregnant clients. Aromatherapy in midwifery is by far the most popular course of all those we offer and I have been invited to many maternity units, both in the United Kingdom and overseas, to help them incorporate aromatherapy and massage into their care of women. The interest in complementary therapies during pregnancy and labour has increased considerably, even in the last five years, and, as you will see in Chapter 1, the number of women accessing therapists or using natural remedies at home, including aromatherapy oils, has grown phenomenally.

Unfortunately, this has brought with it some new problems, mainly as a result of the misconception that natural remedies, including aromatherapy oils, are safer than conventional medical options. The number of women misguidedly using essential oils inappropriately has risen to almost epidemic proportions. Alongside this, the rate of unforeseen events occurring in pregnancy or labour has grown, with women being admitted to hospital with preterm contractions or excessive uterine activity at term, leading to fetal distress (see Chapter 4). Discussions via my LinkedIn group – Complementary Therapies in Maternity Care – indicate that similar problems are occurring in many other countries. This has led to midwives being largely unprepared to advise women on the safety aspects, notably because the subject is not seen as a priority in midwifery pre-registration education and often focuses only on the benefits of the therapies when included in post-registration continuing professional development.

I believe fervently that there is an urgent need for the whole subject of 'complementary therapies' to be included in midwifery training and ongoing education, but we are still some way off from that becoming the norm. It is for this reason that I wanted to write a new textbook on aromatherapy for midwives and other health professionals who work with pregnant and labouring women. In this new book I have applied aromatherapy practice more closely to physiology, reinforced the messages about safety and professional accountability and have drawn on the most recent research I could find to support the claims made for aromatherapy. The detail is considerably greater than in my first two books and I hope it is in keeping with contemporary healthcare practice and education.

My aim, obviously, is to encourage the development of aromatherapy (and other complementary therapies) as a significant subject with which midwives and maternity workers must become familiar, so that they can promote the benefits of aromatherapy and massage in pregnancy and birth, whilst being aware of the safety and professional aspects. I would like to leave a legacy for midwifery in which the subject becomes a standard component of learning, even though not all practitioners may wish to use it in their own practice. We all have a lot of educating of women to do. By writing this book, I hope to help midwives and others to achieve that aim. I hope you enjoy reading it and find it useful in your practice.

Chapter 1

Complementary Therapies in Pregnancy and Childbirth

This chapter includes discussion on:
- introduction to complementary therapies
- aromatherapy as a holistic therapy
- incidence of use of complementary therapies in pregnancy and childbirth
- midwives' use of complementary therapies
- aromatherapy to normalise birth
- dissent for complementary therapies.

Introduction

Aromatherapy is one of many different therapies classified as 'complementary' to mainstream healthcare. Whilst most complementary therapies sit outside conventional health service provision, aromatherapy, and its associated therapy, massage, is increasingly being used by midwives and nurses, and by other health professionals, such as physiotherapists, to enhance normal practice.

In the past 30 years, there has been tremendous growth in the use of complementary therapies and natural remedies, with corresponding attempts by the UK government and the European Union to regulate and control it. In the early 1980s, these therapies were considered very much as 'alternatives' or even 'fringe' medicine. In the 1990s, following a government working party investigating their rise in popularity amongst the general public, they were referred to as 'non-conventional', and it was not until 2000 that the whole system became known as 'complementary and alternative medicine' or CAM.

Complementary therapies incorporate strategies which can be used as an *adjunct to* conventional healthcare, whereas 'alternative' therapies are used *instead of*, although this latter term is less frequently used now. A more commonly used contemporary term is 'integrative medicine', implying that the therapies are integrated into mainstream healthcare, when they may be provided by complementary therapists working alongside orthodox healthcare professionals. For example, many doctors now accept the use of complementary therapies for patients receiving treatment for life-limiting illnesses, such as cancer or Parkinson's disease, as a means of boosting physical and emotional wellbeing (Ben Arye *et al.* 2014; Chen *et al.* 2015; Rao *et al.* 2015). When integrated into biomedicine, the use of the term 'integrative' medicine implies person-centred care (Roberti di Sarsina and Tassinari 2015), possibly to compensate for the shortcomings of conventional healthcare systems in the Western world (Bataller-Sifre and Bataller-Alberola 2015). In the context of pregnancy, labour and the puerperium, all therapies should be *complementary* to standard maternity care, even when they are provided by independent practitioners. When aromatherapy is used by midwives and other maternity care providers within normal antenatal, intrapartum or postnatal care, this is truly integrated, as it is used alongside and in combination with standard care and treatment.

In 2000, the House of Lords published the results of another working party which had examined complementary and alternative medicine, in response to increasing public use and concerns regarding the training and preparation of practitioners, regulation of the therapies and the degree of research evidence to support safety and effectiveness. This sixth report from the Science and Technology Committee (House of Lords 2000) classified the main therapies in use in the United Kingdom at this time into three main groups according to their supposed 'status'. The publication of the report caused considerable controversy and triggered furious debate amongst complementary healthcare practitioners because there was no real consensus of opinion on the classifications. It was generally considered, by many in the complementary healthcare arena, to be a huge political exercise, with those therapies with the largest organisations, especially therapies which were also often practised by medical doctors whose political influence is substantial, being classified in Group 1 and known as the 'Big Five'. Therapies used alongside other healthcare practices, often with shorter training periods and – allegedly – less evidence were allocated to Group 2 as 'supportive' therapies. Traditional therapies from outside the Western world were relegated to Group 3, partly because any herbal medicines brought into the United Kingdom for use by these practitioners could not be adequately monitored or controlled by the UK authorities. Also included in Group 3 were any alternative (i.e. non-medical) methods of diagnosis. Everything else was discarded into an unclassified group. Although the House of Lords report was published in 2000 and is largely outdated, its findings remain contentious but nothing has since replaced it. It is therefore useful, for the sake of reference, to include the classifications here (see Table 1.1).

Table 1.1 Classification of complementary and alternative therapies (according to the House of Lords Report 2000)

GROUP	GROUP 1	GROUP 2	GROUP 3
Definition	**Discrete therapies** considered therapeutic modalities in their own right, with recognised training and continuing professional development (CPD), formal regulation and good evidence base	**Supportive therapies** used in conjunction with other therapies or conventional healthcare; less robust education, regulation and evidence base	**Alternative therapies** with little requirement for formal education, no formal regulation and very poor evidence base
Therapies	Acupuncture (Western) Chiropractic Herbal medicine Homeopathy Osteopathy	Alexander technique Aromatherapy Bach flower remedies Counselling Hydrotherapy Hypnotherapy Massage Nutrition therapies Reflexology Reiki Shiatsu Stress management Yoga	**Group 3a Traditional systems of medicine** (e.g. Ayurveda, Chinese, *kampo*, Tibetan medicine, etc.) **Group 3b Alternative diagnostic techniques** (e.g. iridology, kinesiology, Kirlian photography, radionics, etc.)

The term 'CAM' is usually used by doctors who practise modalities such as acupuncture or homeopathy alongside their normal practice. In some respects this is political nomenclature, implying as it does that certain therapies with well-defined education requirements, regulation and a sound evidence-base fit into the medical model, ostensibly raising their credibility. Some therapies, such as herbal medicine, have raised their profile through degree-level education and voluntary self-regulation. Two therapies in particular, osteopathy and chiropractic, are no longer considered 'complementary' but as professions 'supplementary to medicine' and now fall outside the principle group of therapies by virtue of statutory regulation in 1993 and 1994, respectively. Strategies practised by nurses, midwives, physiotherapists and, of course, complementary practitioners – notably those considered 'supportive' rather than as standalone modalities, tend to be known as 'therapies' rather than 'medicine'. 'Traditional' medicine, classified in Group 3, is usually taken to mean therapies and remedies used in cultures which adhere to the old ways of healing, notably amongst Asian, African and South American peoples.

There are in fact several hundred therapies under the umbrella term of 'complementary therapies' although some of these are deviations from, or new developments of, others – for example, cranio-sacral therapy is an adaptation from osteopathy. Some therapies are much more acceptable to the general public and the medical professions, whilst others remain very much on the 'fringe', including many alternative treatments for cancer, some of which are highly suspect and even dangerous. Each therapy has its own distinct knowledge base, skills, mechanism of action, indications, precautions, contraindications and side-effects, and, for some, an increasing amount of research evidence. Therapies may involve manual techniques, such as massage, osteopathy, chiropractic, reflexology or shiatsu. They may be energy therapies – for example, acupuncture, reiki or homeopathy – or psychological therapies including hypnosis and neuro-linguistic programming.

The term 'natural remedies' applies to any substances which are not commercially prepared drugs. This includes herbal medicines and aromatherapy oils, which act pharmacologically, as well as energy-based medicines, such as homeopathy and flower remedies (e.g. Bach and Australian Bush essences). Remedies made from indigenous plants used in Chinese medicine, Indian Ayurveda, Japanese *kampo* and other traditional forms of medicine also come under the umbrella term of natural remedies, as do nutritional supplements and herbal teas when intended for use as pharmacologically active therapeutic agents. It is interesting to note that the term 'non-pharmacological' therapies is occasionally used erroneously to indicate natural remedy modalities which are not part of mainstream medicine, despite several having a direct pharmacological action, including aromatherapy and herbal medicine (see Table 1.2).

Table 1.2 Classification by mechanism of action of complementary therapies commonly used in the United Kingdom (2016)

MANUAL/TOUCH THERAPIES	PHARMACOLOGICAL THERAPIES	ENERGY-BASED THERAPIES	PSYCHOLOGICAL THERAPIES
Acupuncture	Aromatherapy	Acupuncture	Acupuncture
Aromatherapy	Herbal medicine	Aromatherapy	Aromatherapy
Bowen technique	Nutritional	Flower remedies	Biofeedback
Chiropractic	therapies	(e.g. Bach/	Hypnotherapy/
Cranio-sacral		Bush/Orchid)	Hypnosis
therapy		Homeopathy	Massage
Massage		Kinesiology	Neuro-linguistic
Osteopathy		Reflexology	programming
Reflexology		Reiki/Spiritual	Reflexology
Shiatsu/		healing	Shiatsu/
Acupressure		Shiatsu/	Acupressure
		Acupressure	

Aromatherapy as a holistic therapy

The focus of all complementary therapies is the concept of 'holism' in which the client is viewed as a whole person, with their physical, mental and spiritual conditions being inter-linked. This is often referred to as the 'mind-body-spirit' approach and is very different from the conventional reductionist medical approach which divides healthcare into specialisms which isolate one part from another, rather like an engine to be dismantled, repaired and reassembled. It is, of course, known that there is a strong link between the physical body and the emotions or mind, not least in terms of the physical effects which can occur during periods of severe stress.

What is less well acknowledged is the concept of spirituality. The spirit is often referred to as the life force which drives us, or the 'breath' of the soul. One's life force can be greatly influenced by thoughts and feelings, with emotions such as happiness and joy keeping the spirit vibrant, and those such as anger and fear threatening to suppress the human spirit. Much of complementary medicine is based on some of these somewhat nebulous and esoteric concepts which are not easily understood, at least in developed Western cultures where everything is supported by factual information and research evidence. There is increasing interest amongst clinical practitioners such as nurses and midwives in the notion of spirituality (Caldeira *et al.* 2015; Foster 2006; Perriam 2015), although this is sometimes misinterpreted as meaning solely religious differences (Cullen 2015). In the maternity arena, spirituality is often discussed in relation to grief, perhaps after stillbirth and, more recently, to finding a 'sacred space' during labour, particularly at the moment of birth (Crowther 2013).

Aromatherapy is said to be a holistic or complementary therapy which affects body, mind and spirit. When essential oils are administered via massage, aromatherapy is also a manual therapy with direct effects on physical structures such as muscles, joints, the lymphatics and the skin. There are many different styles of massage, including traditional Swedish massage, lymphatic drainage, intuitive or formally structured styles, light-touch massage, or deep touch such as rolfing. Other manual modalities may be added into the massage, with or without essential oils – for example, reflexology, shiatsu or acupressure. Aromatherapy is also a natural remedy system in which the essential oils, once absorbed into the body, act pharmacologically, either systemically as on the circulation and blood pressure, or on specific organs, depending on the administration techniques and specific oils used. It is also said to be a spiritual therapy in that the aromas and the chemicals within the essential oils can contribute to an overall sense of wellbeing, affecting body, mind and spirit. The essential oils have been shown to have psycho-emotional effects, plus the relaxation impact of massage makes aromatherapy a dynamic therapy for mental and emotional wellbeing – a true holistic therapy. In addition, a major feature of aromatherapy and other complementary modalities is the impact of the client–therapist relationship, which enhances the spiritual benefits of the treatment.

Incidence of use of complementary therapies in pregnancy and childbirth

In Westernised countries, it has been estimated that at least one in three of the general population now uses complementary medicine, although a UK study (Hunt *et al.* 2010) suggested that this may have risen in recent years, with 44% of the general public using therapies, notably massage, aromatherapy and acupuncture. Women are more likely to use complementary therapies than men (Hunt *et al.* 2010) and, as may be expected, young men in their late teens and early twenties are least likely of all groups to access any form of healthcare (Jain and Astin 2001). However, specific survey results are mostly outdated and more recent studies tend to focus on the prevalence of use amongst specific groups of the population – for example, amongst cancer sufferers. Unresolved pain and other subjective symptoms may also lead people to consider complementary medicine (Sharpe *et al.* 2015), particularly for those with chronic or life-limiting conditions such as breast cancer (Chandwani *et al.* 2014).

The number of pregnant women accessing complementary therapies or self-administering natural remedies has grown considerably in the last 5–10 years. Many women have used complementary therapies before becoming pregnant, either for general wellbeing and relaxation for themselves and their families, or for alternative treatment of a specific condition. Aromatherapy oils in particular are frequently self-administered at home for problems such as dysmenorrhoea or insomnia, or simply for general relaxation – for example by adding them to the bath water or for use in vaporisers.

Some couples may consult independent therapists prior to conception, especially for fertility issues. The fast pace of life today means that many women (and men) are stressed more than ever before, and the economic need, in most families, for both partners to work leaves very little 'me time' for relaxation. Not only has this resulted in women leaving it late to start a family, but stress and increasing age have led to more difficulties in conceiving. Having benefited from complementary therapies before conception, many women continue to access them once pregnant, or they may use natural remedies at home. Increasingly, pregnant women request information and advice on natural ways to deal with the discomforts they experience, not least because they are warned that they should, wherever possible, avoid taking medication. Added to this is the shortage of midwifery staff and time constraints, which means that women may feel unable to discuss minor anxieties with their midwives at their antenatal appointments. Expectant mothers may decide to consult complementary practitioners for relaxation and ready access to spending time with a professional who will listen to their worries, as well as seeking treatment for the various discomforts of pregnancy such as backache or sickness. Later, women may wish to be accompanied in labour by an independent therapist, or a doula or birth supporter who uses complementary therapies. Further, many women seem desperate to expedite labour and avoid induction, and frequently use natural remedies, often inappropriately, to trigger contractions.

The incidence of complementary therapy use in pregnancy is estimated to be anything from 6–91% (Bishop et al. 2011; Frawley et al. 2014; Hall, Griffiths and McKenna 2011; Pallivalapila et al. 2015), although most of these surveys relate more to the self-use of natural remedies than to consulting practitioners for manual and psychological therapies. In the United States, Holden et al. (2015) obtained statistics on over 10,000 pregnant women and found that more than 30% used complementary therapies, often without informing their maternity caregivers. A large study across 23 countries in Europe, North and South America and Australia (Kennedy et al. 2013) showed an average use of herbal medicines of 28.9%, with wide variations between countries, while Sibbritt et al. (2014) found that around 15% self-prescribed aromatherapy oils for use at home.

Use of natural remedies appears to increase as pregnancy progresses and women prepare for birth (Bishop et al. 2011). Unsurprisingly, their use declines postnatally, presumably because women are more focused on the baby than themselves (Birdee et al. 2014), although some turn to herbal remedies to aid lactation (Sim et al. 2013). As with the American study, other researchers have revealed that only about half of those using complementary therapies inform their maternity care providers (Strouss et al. 2014; Warriner, Bryan and Brown 2014). Interestingly, in an Italian study, Trabace et al. (2015) found that 72% of women did inform their doctors about their use of herbal remedies, but this may reflect a greater acceptance of self-administration in this part of Europe and a greater use of natural remedies by midwives in Italy. However, the general trend towards covert use in most countries may be because women do not think it is necessary or relevant to their care to inform their midwives or obstetricians (Babycentre 2011). There is also a major lack of understanding of the potential risks of using complementary therapies during pregnancy and childbirth, particularly as women are almost universally more likely to access the Internet, television and magazines or ask friends and family for information rather than referring to health professionals (Bond et al. 2014; Hall et al. 2011; Pallivalapila et al. 2015; Strouss et al. 2014). Studies on the use of herbal medicines in particular have found adverse effects from ingestion of chamomile, ginger and sweet fennel, including preterm labour and low birthweight or reduced length or skull circumference in neonates (Trabace *et al.* 2015).

It is worth considering which women use complementary therapies during pregnancy. A Canadian study (Feijen-de Jong *et al.* 2015) found that those with private health insurance, or women who had had a previous poor experience of conventional maternity care, often chose to consult complementary practitioners. Certainly, many women have sufficient disposable income to be able to choose to access complementary therapies for relaxation, particularly when the conventional maternity services are stretched to their limit, causing many women to feel that midwives do not have time to discuss worries with them. Women are often very anxious, even without previous traumatic experiences of pregnancy and birth, and consulting a complementary practitioner may be seen as a compensation for the perceived paucity of quality maternity services.

The level of education appears to be significant in decision-making about complementary therapies (Hunt *et al.* 2010), particularly university-level education (Pallivalapila *et al.* 2015), although there is an almost universal lack of knowledge about the apparent safety of natural remedies (Warriner *et al.* 2014). Many women with a good knowledge of how to live healthily frequently use complementary medicine, although Feijen-de Jong *et al.* (2015) showed that those in their study who smoked or drank alcohol regularly were also seen to seek alternatives to mainstream care. Other researchers suggest that complementary therapy use aids relaxation and empowers women, helping them to maintain control over their bodies; indeed, it can have a transformational effect on the mother and her attitude to pregnancy and motherhood (Mitchell 2014, 2015). Frawley *et al.* (2015) found that women with anxiety commonly turned to herbal remedies, particularly for insomnia and fatigue, while Pallivalapila *et al.* (2015) showed that women with a personal or family use of complementary medicine were the most common users.

Expectant mothers in many countries around the world use indigenous herbal remedies, including aromatherapy oils, and although the specific remedies may vary, the problems for maternity professionals are much the same: inappropriate use causing complications and the failure of women to inform their caregivers. In Africa, at least 50% of women resort to natural methods of dealing with pregnancy issues or to induce miscarriage or prepare for birth (Bayisa, Tatiparthi and Mulisa 2014; Constant *et al.* 2014; Yemele *et al.* 2015). This is often compounded by the spiritual nature of traditional medicine, including its association in many African countries with witchcraft. In the Middle East, around 26–30% of expectant mothers appear to use herbal medicines, influenced by parity, geographical location and education (Sattari *et al.* 2012), whereas in parts of South America the incidence of use appears to be around 19% (Bercaw, Maheshwari and Sangi-Haghpeykar 2010), although this also varies between countries.

Sibbritt *et al.* (2014) specifically explored the prevalence of use of aromatherapy in pregnancy and found that 15.2% of expectant mothers self-administered essential oils, notably for hayfever or allergies or, rather worryingly, if they had a urinary tract infection. The authors expressed concern about this. They stated that midwives and doctors must be alert to the fact that women may be using essential oils and should initiate discussion with them about the potential risks. In Bishop *et al.*'s (2011) Bristol survey, less than 1% of women were found to use aromatherapy; homeopathic remedies were much more prevalent, but this may have been due to a geographical focus on homeopathy as a result of the original siting of one of the United Kingdom's National Health Service (NHS) homeopathic hospitals (now closed). Furthermore, news at the time of writing suggests that homeopathic remedies, which have always been available on the NHS since its inception, may soon no longer be available via NHS prescription (BBC News 2015).

However, the prevalence of use of complementary therapies in general may be far greater than current studies suggest. It would be valuable to conduct a UK-wide survey to discover the true incidence of antenatal and intrapartum use of aromatherapy. Warriner *et al.* (2014) undertook a study in one UK NHS maternity unit in which interviews were conducted with pregnant women about their use of herbal remedies. Their findings bear out those of other studies around the world, in which women see herbal medicine as outside the mainstream and part of an empowering holistic approach to self-care, used partly due to dissatisfaction with conventional maternity services and partly because they believe, incorrectly, that natural remedies are safer than medical drugs.

As stated previously, very few women inform their midwife or doctor about their use of natural remedies (Warriner *et al.* 2014), but anecdotal evidence indicates a phenomenal use of aromatherapy oils and other plant substances, especially in relation to initiating contractions around term. Numerous situations have been reported to this author in which women have been found to have used excessively large doses of essential oils. One of the commonest oils used appears to be clary sage, which is useful for midwives to use as a post-dates pregnancy treatment (see Chapters 5 and 6), but some women have been found to administer it neat onto the abdomen from as early as 30 weeks gestation, subsequently experiencing threatened preterm labour. The general public is largely unaware of the possible risks of essential oils and there is the common misconception that these remedies are safe because they are natural. Consumers (and many professionals) fail to understand that essential oils contain chemicals, that the mechanism of action of the chemical constituents in the essential oils is pharmacological and that there are certain women who should refrain from using the oils in the preconception, antenatal, intrapartum and breastfeeding periods (see Chapter 4).

These figures suggest that midwives should make a point of asking women, at the time of the booking history, about their use of complementary therapies and natural remedies in order to avoid the risks of inadvertent adverse effects of the oils or the possibility of interactions with medications. Questions may need to be asked again in the third trimester, since many women often only start considering the use of natural strategies as they approach labour – for example, the popular herbal remedy, raspberry leaf tea. It is also important to ascertain on meeting a mother in early labour whether she has yet used any natural remedies, perhaps for pain relief or relaxation, or intends to do so as the labour progresses.

Midwives' use of complementary therapies

In response to the demand from expectant mothers for information on complementary therapies and natural remedies, midwives and other maternity care providers, such as doulas, antenatal teachers and other birth workers, have become increasingly interested in the subject. This author has been working in the specialist field of maternity-related complementary medicine for over 30 years and has witnessed considerable growth in the number of midwives and doulas wanting to study complementary therapies, including aromatherapy, massage, reflexology, hypnosis ('hypno-birthing') and acupuncture. Aromatherapy is by far the most popular therapy and, for midwives wanting to implement complementary therapies into their practice, one of the easiest. Many NHS hospitals in the United Kingdom, as well as maternity units overseas, are encouraging midwives to develop the knowledge and skills to use aromatherapy for women, especially in labour (see Resources section for information on training courses).

Conversely, many midwives and doulas take it upon themselves to recommend complementary therapies without any real understanding of the safety or professional accountability issues. Stewart *et al.* (2014) demonstrated that around 30% of midwives offer advice on the subject, notably those who are personal users. In Australia, Hall, Griffiths and McKenna (2013a) found that midwives working with women who are keen to use complementary therapies attempt to act as their advocate by supporting their choices, whilst being mindful of safety. However, a previous study by the same team (Hall, Griffiths and McKenna 2012; Hall, McKenna and Griffiths 2012b) found that many midwives were conscious of opposition or scepticism from their medical colleagues, leading them to use a variety of strategies to avoid conflict, including asking women not to disclose to the doctor that the midwife was their source of information.

Adams *et al.* (2015) suggest that communication between pregnant women and their caregivers, as well as between conventional and complementary practitioners, must be improved in order to avoid some of the clinical problems which can occur from inappropriate use. This requires midwives and obstetricians to be more aware of the risks as well as the benefits and to engage in research studies to demonstrate both safety and effectiveness. Midwives, in particular, need adequate education and professional guidance so that they are better equipped, and more confident, to provide accurate, comprehensive and evidence-based support to their clients (Hall, Griffiths and McKenna 2013b; Tiran 2004, 2010a, 2011a). Making the subject a compulsory part of the midwifery pre-registration curriculum, as seen in some medical and pharmacy training programmes (Bailey *et al.* 2015; Esposito, Bystrek and Klein 2014), could contribute to a greater understanding of safety, more facilitative attitudes and an increased desire to incorporate aspects of complementary therapies into conventional practice (Tiran 2011a, 2011b).

Aromatherapy to normalise birth

The nurturing power of aromatherapy and massage fits well with the philosophy of midwifery care. Not only do they offer the mother ways to aid relaxation and ease pain, but they also help midwives to return to being 'with woman', and to engage in those traditional aspects of care which are so much a part of the human experience of being pregnant and giving birth. Essential oils and more highly refined skills in massage techniques provide caregivers with new tools to add to their existing strategies, empowering both the mothers and themselves.

Perhaps most significant, is the value of any relaxation therapies in reducing stress, tension and anxiety and the impact this can have on normalising childbirth (Bastard and Tiran 2006). Dhany, Mitchell and Foy (2012) found that intrapartum aromatherapy reduced the need for analgesia such as pethidine and epidural, and where standard pain relief was required, women were better able to cope just using inhalational analgesia or transcutaneous electrical nerve stimulation (TENS). Similar findings were obtained by Burns *et al.* (2000), who also noted the decrease in use of oxytocics. Using aromatherapy and massage in labour is known to reduce cortisol and anxiety (McNabb *et al.* 2006) and improves maternal satisfaction with the birth experience (Mortazavi *et al.* 2012), thus facilitating oxytocin release and enabling women to labour more normally (see also Chapter 2 for more discussion on the benefits of massage in pregnancy and birth).

The need to reduce intervention has fuelled a desire amongst midwives to find new ways of helping women during pregnancy and labour in order to facilitate normal progress. An average 25% of births in the United Kingdom are now by Caesarean section (Birth Choice UK 2014), which is known to contribute to avoidable safety incidents (King's Fund 2009). Induction of labour accounts for around 23% of births, with rates rising year on year, yet induction, specifically for post-dates pregnancy as opposed to any medical or obstetric indication, increases the likelihood of requiring a Caesarean (Jacquemyn *et al.* 2012). Women opting for private maternity care are shown to have an even greater chance of having an operative delivery than those receiving publically funded care (Dahlen *et al.* 2012). Caesareans consume enormous resources: in 2009, the cost of a normal birth in the United Kingdom averaged £749, whereas Caesareans cost more than double at £1701 (NHS Institute for Innovation and Improvement 2009). To put this into context, in a maternity unit with 6000 births per annum, reducing a 25% Caesarean rate to 20% would save at least £285,000 annually; nationally this could save the NHS over £33 million a year! In addition, the long-term sequelae of operative delivery, and the psycho-social impact on the mother and family consume further resources which are more difficult to estimate since they may come from other clinical budgets.

However, the context in which midwives respond to women's demands for complementary therapies has changed in the last decade. Whilst midwives' interests may have sprung initially from a desire to find new 'tools' with which to care for women holistically, it could be argued that women are now seeking complementary therapies because they want better service during pregnancy and birth. There is so much dissatisfaction with the maternity services that perhaps what all women actually want is simply to have a caring competent midwife (or other practitioner) who treats them in a way which focuses on the huge importance of this life event for each woman. Women want continuity of carer; they do not overtly request complementary therapies from their midwife. Further, whilst women are accessing complementary therapies elsewhere (i.e. outside the mainstream maternity services), midwives may be at risk of misinterpreting this as a demand for complementary therapies to be provided by midwives. This has led, in some maternity units, to midwives and their managers attempting to implement several complementary therapies into care provision. However, this tactic is likely to fragment care even further, since it would be impossible for all midwives to be trained to provide all therapies, thus requiring a mother to be treated with complementary therapies by a midwife who is not her named midwife. It must also be remembered that any intervention in a normal physio-psycho-social life event is an intervention, not least the use of complementary therapies which are outside normal service provision. However, in defence of aromatherapy, this is one of the therapies which can more easily be incorporated into care by all members of the midwifery team, using a formulaic approach to provide a limited service, perhaps only in labour (see Chapter 5 on implementation of aromatherapy).

Conversely, massage has traditionally been an instinctive part of the repertoire of techniques used by midwives when caring for women in labour. Nicholas Culpeper, the celebrated 17th-century herbalist, advised that 'if travel [labour] be hard, anoint the belly and sides with oyl of sweet almonds, lilies and sweet wine' (Thomas 1993). The pioneer of natural childbirth, Grantly Dick-Read, advocated pain-relieving labour massage by birth attendants in 1933 (Dick-Read 2013). Kerstin Uvnäs-Moberg (2011), in her book *The Oxytocin Factor*, emphasises the benefits of massage in activating what she terms the 'calm and connection' system. Adding the use of fragrant essential oils, known for their various physiological properties which arise from the chemical constituents, can aid a woman's progress in labour by keeping her relaxed and facilitating the production of oxytocin. Whilst there is no guarantee that aromatherapy and massage will avoid intervention, it encourages the mother to focus on being in tune with her body, and the attention and individualised care from the midwife will add to the mother's sense of wellbeing.

Several authorities and national documents have expressed concern about the levels of intervention in childbirth, and support the use of any strategies which may contribute to a more normal birth. The King's Fund's report (2009) on safety incidents ('near misses') in maternity care directly attributed these events to the inappropriately high levels of medical intervention and suggested that litigation costs could be reduced by returning to a more physiological approach to childbirth. The NHS Institute for Innovation and Improvement (2009) also focused on public health issues in its document on High Impact Actions for Nursing and Midwifery, suggesting an urgent need to reduce interventions in childbirth by whatever means possible. In 2014 the Royal College of Midwives launched its Better Births Campaign, with an introductory webinar by Professor Soo Downe, who states that:

> If routine interventions are eliminated for healthy women and babies, resources will be freed up for the extra staff, treatments and interventions [for] when a labouring woman and her baby actually need help. This will ensure optimal outcomes for all women and babies, and sustainable maternity care provision overall. (Downe 2014)

Using massage and aromatherapy during the first stage of labour can help to promote a peaceful birth environment, which in turn allows the mother to labour more productively, thus reducing the need for epidural anaesthesia or for the augmentation of labour. Enabling and empowering the mother to believe in herself by receiving nurturing touch and massage and through attention to creating a calming birth environment enhances her feeling of control, her sense of satisfaction and her belief in her ability to give birth to her baby naturally.

Dissent for complementary therapies

It is reassuring that attention is now being given to reducing medical intervention in childbirth, and to appreciating the value of complementary therapies. The broad area of complementary and alternative medicine is not, however, without its critics. Even where tacit approval appears to be given, it is usually with a strongly worded proviso to use caution and to seek medical advice, together with concern being expressed about the lack of evidence. Even though it is largely true that there *is* a need for more research, it is unhelpful to make a blanket statement about 'lack of evidence', especially given that many aspects of conventional healthcare have been introduced without adequate prior evaluation. Further, it is highly unlikely that many medical practitioners will be sufficiently cognisant of the risks of complementary therapies and natural remedies to be able to advise patients appropriately.

The NHS Choices website (2015a) focuses on the relaxation element of many therapies and the inherent placebo effect. Site users are directed to the guidelines produced by the National Institute for Health and Care Excellence (NICE). On its online page entitled 'Are complementary therapies safe in pregnancy?' the NHS Choices website (2015b) again takes a very cautious view, suggesting, appropriately, that women should avoid any unnecessary medicines or treatments when pregnant. However, the validity of this statement in respect of all medicines and medical techniques during pregnancy is overshadowed by the repetitive statement about lack of evidence for complementary therapies. It is also interesting to note that, whilst the Complementary and Natural Healthcare Council (CNHC) is mentioned as one of the voluntary regulatory bodies for practitioners (and is the one which is generally considered to be most closely aligned with the NHS), there is no direct link to the CNHC website, there being instead a link to another voluntary organisation, the Institute for Complementary and Natural Medicine (ICNM), which is not as active as the CNHC. Further, it has not been acknowledged that there are numerous charitable organisations providing registration for complementary therapists, plus indemnity insurance and other professional services. Identifying one organisation in particular on a major national public website is monopolistic and biased.

The NICE guidelines on antenatal care (NICE 2014a) have very conflicting and incorrect statements regarding complementary therapies in pregnancy. On the one hand, they state that care should be woman-centred and facilitate informed decision-making, suggesting that those women wishing to use complementary therapies should be helped to do so safely and appropriately. However, whilst they emphasise that care must be based on currently available evidence, they fail to recognise that some of their statements about complementary therapies in the guideline are incorrect. The advice states that 'pregnant women should be informed that few complementary therapies have been established as being safe and effective during pregnancy. Women should not assume that such therapies are safe and they should be used as little as possible during pregnancy' (NICE 2014a, para 1.3.6.1).

The revised intrapartum guidelines (NICE 2014b), whilst sanctioning the use of massage in labour, go one step further in generally rejecting complementary therapies, by stating, in respect of pain relief in the latent phase of labour: 'Do not offer or advise aromatherapy, yoga or acupressure for pain relief during the latent first stage of labour. If a woman wants to use any of these techniques, respect her wishes' (p.332, clause 5.2.8.40). This is unhelpful in the extreme when women are frequently using or asking about complementary therapies for labour and midwives are attempting to implement aromatherapy and other therapies into their care of women in labour. It is especially galling when some large-scale (but, unfortunately, not all randomised controlled) studies have shown the benefits of aromatherapy in reducing fear, pain, analgesia and oxytocic use and improving maternal satisfaction (Burns *et al.* 2000, 2007). Similarly, in relation to established labour, the guidelines on pain relief state: 'Do not offer acupuncture, acupressure or hypnosis, but do not prevent women who wish to use these techniques from doing so' (NICE 2014b, p.365, clause 8.3.7.8.72).

It is evident that members of the working parties on these two NICE guidelines have no real knowledge or understanding of complementary therapies. Indeed, in the 'common disorders of pregnancy' section of the antenatal care guideline, the recommendation to advise ginger to all women with sickness is based purely on evidence of effectiveness and not on the slightly more obscure, but nevertheless relevant and increasing evidence on safety – or more significantly, the risks of ginger (Tiran 2012). Furthermore, the guidelines advocate several strategies which actually fall into the category of 'complementary therapies', such as acupressure wristbands for sickness and massage for backache. Although the NICE publications are intended primarily as guidance – and there are many other recommendations which have been challenged by midwives – some maternity units view them as policy, which leads to difficulties when midwives wish to implement these strategies into their care of women. It also perpetuates the disparaging attitude held about complementary therapies by some midwives and doctors, which does nothing to support women and risks the covert use of potentially hazardous substances in pregnancy or labour.

Cochrane reviews, on the other hand, sometimes conflict with the NICE guidelines, although the standard conclusion to most systematic reviews is that further research is necessary. Smith, Collins and Crowther (2011) found only two randomised controlled studies of aromatherapy for pain management in labour, while Jones *et al.* (2012) found evidence of good effectiveness for epidural anaesthesia, or spinal anaesthesia and inhalational analgesia, possible effectiveness for water immersion, massage, acupuncture and relaxation techniques, and insufficient evidence for aromatherapy, hypnosis, biofeedback, TENS and sterile water injections. More positively, Liddle and Pennick's (2015) recent systematic review of low back and pelvic pain in pregnancy found good evidence to support the use of acupuncture, osteopathy, chiropractic and cranio-sacral therapy. Similarly, Coyle, Smith and Peat (2012) gave a cautious welcome to the use of moxibustion for turning a breech to cephalic presentation. Although there was little evidence of its direct success, they did acknowledge that it may be useful, in conjunction with acupuncture, in increasing the success rate of external cephalic version and reducing the need for oxytocics or Caesarean section.

Conclusion

Aromatherapy is one of many different complementary therapies which may be useful in maternity care. However, whilst many pregnant women are keen to use it, either by consulting a practitioner or through self-administration of the essential oils, provision of aromatherapy is not yet universal throughout the maternity services. There is emerging evidence that using strategies which contribute to normalising birth can reduce interventions, complications and long-term sequelae and improve maternal satisfaction, and there are examples of maternity units in which midwives have implemented aromatherapy very successfully, despite dissent from NICE and some other authorities. Whilst there remains a need for further research evidence, there is an increasing amount of investigation into both individual essential oils and the 'package' of care in which aromatherapy and massage are used (see Chapter 3). This, then, is the context in which midwives and other maternity professionals must work to include aromatherapy in their practice. Midwives are keen to use aromatherapy and other complementary therapies and can demonstrate the benefits of incorporating them into standard care, but must take care to work within 'the system' when implementing aromatherapy in their practice.

Chapter 2

Principles and Practice of Aromatherapy

This chapter includes discussion on:

- definitions of aromatherapy
- history of aromatherapy
- contemporary regulation of aromatherapy
- European Union (EU) Directives
- what essential oils are
- extraction of essential oils from plants
- purchasing quality essential oils for aromatherapy practice
- storage of essential oils
- dosages in maternity aromatherapy
- blending of essential oils
- methods of administration of essential oils:
  - administration of essential oils via the respiratory tract: inhalation
  - administration of essential oils via the skin: massage
  - administration of essential oils via the skin: in water
  - principles of administration of aromatherapy in pregnancy and childbirth.

Definitions of aromatherapy

Aromatherapy is considered to be an artistic and scientific modality based on the principle that highly concentrated aromatic essential oils extracted from different parts of plants are administered in various ways for their therapeutic purposes in order to enhance health and wellbeing.

There are, in fact, three different 'sciences' within the overall umbrella term of aromatherapy. First, aromachology, or psycho-aromatherapy, is based on the impact of the aromas of the essential oils on the brain, notably the limbic system, and the effects of those aromas on emotions and feelings. Second, aromatology is concerned with the internal use of essential oils (gastrointestinal, *per vaginam, per rectum*), administered as medicines, as practised in parts of Europe outside the United Kingdom, normally by medically qualified physicians and medical herbalists. In this case, the term '*aromatology*' is misleading as the aromas have virtually no effect once the oil has passed via the mucosa.

Third, aromatherapy, as defined by the US Sense of Smell Institute, involves the therapeutic use of the aromas of essential oils on physical or psychological conditions. This term has, however, been interwoven into a modality in which the method of administration, such as massage, plays a part in the overall therapeutic effect, and many medical authorities deem aromatherapy to have little more than a placebo effect. Indeed, Lis-Balchin (2010) disparages modern UK aromatherapy as insufficiently evidence-based, suggesting that it is often practised by inadequately trained practitioners who purport to apply a scientific approach and who sometimes combine it with 'more dubious alternative disciplines' such as cosmology, crystals and chakra balancing. The fact that most clients consult aromatherapists for 'stress-related' disorders and that any improvement is due largely to an increased sense of relaxation further fuels her disenchantment with contemporary aromatherapy as a clinical modality in the Western world.

Despite Lis-Balchin's somewhat negative perspective on modern therapeutic aromatherapy, this book is concerned with the generally held view of aromatherapy as a healing modality. In maternity care, it offers the possibility of a return to normality in childbirth and enables women to enjoy their experiences of pregnancy, which like so many other situations has become yet another 'medical' condition. (See Chapter 1 for more discussion on the reasons why women seek aromatherapy.)

There is certainly an increasing interest in the stress-reducing impact of aromatherapy amongst conventional healthcare professionals. We know that high levels of stress hormones have adverse effects on health and wellbeing, including impairment of the immune system, greater perception of pain and interference with other endocrinological functions (see Chapter 3). Thus the benefits of a relatively inexpensive, easily administered and generally enjoyable therapy suggest that its value goes beyond the purely scientific evidence currently available. Also, in maternity care, the impact of human touch – in this case, massage – is invaluable in this era of technological intervention, electronic monitoring and staff shortages, providing a much appreciated human interaction. In addition, whether or not aromatherapy works through some placebo effect may not yet be fully understood. However, there is ample evidence that the placebo effect in itself can be beneficial in many medical conditions, and doctors are now encouraged to 'exploit' this in their care and advice to patients (Flaherty, Fitzgibbon and Cantillon 2015). For whatever reason, the interaction between therapist and client, the use of touch, the client's – or the therapist's – belief in the efficacy of the treatment, or some other factor, may give rise to a positive alteration in the wellbeing of the client.

Essential oils contain numerous chemicals which have a range of physical and emotional effects. These chemical constituents work pharmacologically (see Chapter 3), having physiological effects on different organs within the body, as well as psychological effects via the limbic system in the brain. The oils can be applied via the skin as a massage, which is by far the most popular method. Dermal administration can also be achieved by adding the essential oils to water, in the bath, a footbath or spray, or as a compress. Inhalation via the respiratory tract can be used as a specific method of administration in its own right but in the United Kingdom is less commonly used than massage. However, every woman receiving aromatherapy treatment by any other method of administration will also inhale the aromas and she is therefore inhaling the chemicals, which will have a physical and emotional impact – with both positive and potentially negative effects.

Oils can also be administered via the mucus membranes, rectally as suppositories, or vaginally as pessaries, but these methods are not appropriate in pregnancy and birth, and should not be used by midwives, doulas or therapists. Finally, essential oils can be given orally via the gastrointestinal tract, but this method is generally only used by medical practitioners, in those European countries where aromatherapy is incorporated into mainstream medicine, with some essential oils being regulated as prescription-only drugs (aromatology). In the United Kingdom it is not possible to obtain indemnity insurance cover for oral administration unless the practitioner is a fully qualified aromatherapist who has undertaken further study in the gastrointestinal administration of essential oils.

The therapeutic effects of aromatherapy are thought to be achieved through a combination of the physiological action of the chemicals in the essential oils, the method of administration and the psychological impact of the aromas. The practitioner, usually in partnership with the client, chooses appropriate essential oils and a method of administration which best suits the client's condition and smell preferences, with the aim of treating specific issues. Aromatherapy is generally considered relaxing, especially when administered as massage, but essential oils can have numerous other effects. Whilst many essential oils are known to have a relaxant effect, such as lavender (Sayorwan *et al.* 2012), or even sedating – for example, chamomile (Chang and Chen 2015) – others are more stimulating. Examples include the following: peppermint, which stimulates the skin and hair (Oh, Park and Kim 2014); grapefruit, which stimulates the sympathetic nervous system (Nagai *et al.* 2014); and black pepper, a rubefacient (warming) oil affecting the circulation (Butt *et al.* 2013). Essential oils such as clary sage and lavender have been shown to lower the systolic and diastolic blood pressure respectively (Seol *et al.* 2013), whereas others are known to raise it, including rosemary (Fernández, Palomino and Frutos 2014). Several essential oils have been found to relieve pain – for example, lemon (Ikeda, Takasu and Murase 2014) and lavender (Hadi and Hanid 2011).

Many essential oils should not be used in the preconception, antenatal and intrapartum periods. Others should be used with caution or may be contraindicated at certain times during the childbearing period, or for women with particular medical or obstetric conditions. It stands to reason, then, that incorrect or inappropriate treatment may, at the very least, fail to have the desired effects, and may even pose risks to the health and wellbeing of the mother and/or fetus. (See Chapter 4 for more on the safety of aromatherapy in pregnancy and childbirth).

The history of aromatherapy

Plants and plant essences have been used for over 3500 years, both for their perfumes and for their supposed medicinal properties. The term 'aromatherapie' has only been used since the beginning of the 20th century, when the French perfumer and chemist, Gattefossé, coined the phrase, possibly to differentiate the medicinal application of essential oils from their use in perfumery. Aromatherapy is inexorably linked to aromatic herbal medicine, which was often combined with religion, mysticism and magic, and in some cultures this is still the case. For example, the medicinal use of plants in India is thought to date back 5000 years and remains part of Ayurvedic medicine, which is widely practised in modern-day India.

The ancient Egyptians burned incense made from aromatic woods, herbs and spices in honour to their gods. They also used aromatic plant oils to embalm and mummify their dead in preparation for the after-life, as the aromas deodorised the corpses and the chemical constituents in them aided preservation. Common oils used for embalming included frankincense, myrrh, cinnamon, juniper berry and spikenard. The Egyptians also traded in aromatic herbs and spices, particularly frankincense and myrrh, and because demand was greater than supply, the oils commanded prices equivalent to that of gold, gems and other precious metals. Their love of perfumes grew, and in the thousand or so years before the birth of Christ, the Egyptian perfumery industry was considered the finest in the Middle East. Cleopatra is thought to have seduced Mark Anthony with her lavish use of aromatic essences and, allegedly, when Julius Caesar returned home with Cleopatra after conquering Egypt, the crowds were showered with perfume and perfume bottles as a means of showing Caesar's total dominance over Egypt.

As the Egyptian empire declined around 300 BC, Europe became the centre of empirical medicine where new methods were steadily evolving into scientific systems of healing. The Greeks used plant oils as perfumes and medicines, and also as incense in their places of worship. They accumulated knowledge gained from the Egyptians and Indians and recorded this for future generations, particularly around 400 BC at the time of Hippocrates. Hippocrates dismissed the Egyptian theory that illness was caused by supernatural forces and believed that doctors should assess each patient individually for their symptoms in order to make a clinical judgement. He used various therapeutic methods including baths, massage and ingestion of herbs such as fennel, parsley or hypericum, and is said to have documented several hundred herbal medicines during his lifetime.

Later, the Greco-Roman physician, Galen, after whom one of the great cerebral veins is named, documented hundreds of herbal medicines. He was followed by Dioscorides, who compiled a 'materia medica', called *Herbaria*, which detailed hundreds of plants and their medicinal properties. There are also accounts in the historical literature of Roman soldiers benefiting from the therapeutic properties of plants – for example, chewing fennel seeds to suppress hunger as they prepared for battle. Similarly, the Bible has several references to essential oils being used to anoint or massage the feet – Mary Magdalen used spikenard ointment to anoint the feet of Jesus before the Last Supper. Around 1000 AD the Persian, Ibn Sina, known to us as Avicenna, is credited with discovering the method of distillation of essential oils, and he contributed to over 20 authoritative texts on the medicinal properties of plants.

European influences on herbal medicine and aromatherapy developed gradually – the earliest known manuscript of botanical medicines is thought to have been written in Anglo-Saxon times. When the Crusaders returned from the Holy Wars, they brought with them perfumes, fragrant waters and herbal medicines which were previously unknown in Britain, and the use of fragrances and medicinal plants grew. However, during the 13th and 14th centuries in Europe, medicine was almost entirely controlled by the Catholic Church, which believed that illness was a punishment from God. The Black Death decimated the population of Europe and although herbs were used medicinally they could not compete with such a virulent disease. In the 17th century, the renowned herbalist, Nicholas Culpeper, was one of the most influential practitioners of his time and, together with other notable herbalists, left a rich legacy of knowledge which would later be developed by the fragrance and food industries and by the emerging pharmacological profession.

The term '*aromathérapie*' was first used by René Maurice Gattefossé (1881–1950), who studied the medicinal properties of aromatic herbs for many years. His interest arose when he burned his hand in a laboratory accident and plunged his hand into the nearest available liquid, which happened to be essential oil of lavender. He was amazed to find that his hand healed with no pain or infection, no blistering or scarring. He went on to research numerous plant oils and published one of the classic texts on aromatherapy in 1937 (Tisserand 1993). A compatriot of Gattefossé, Jean Valnet, who worked as a surgical assistant in the First World War, used essential oils of chamomile, lemon, thyme and clove to treat gangrenous wounds on the battlefield. On qualifying as a doctor after the war, he continued to use essential oils for medicinal purposes and was the first clinician to use them for psychiatric conditions. His textbook on aromatherapy, written in 1964, was translated into English in 1980, finally putting aromatherapy on the English scene (Valnet 1980).

Aromatherapy as a profession was brought to the United Kingdom in the late 1950s by the Austrian-born biochemist, nurse and cosmetologist, Madame Marguerite Maury, who is credited with developing the addition of essential oils to carrier oils to be used in massage. Unfortunately, in those early days in Britain, aromatherapy became closely aligned to the beauty therapy industry, which could be said to have had a detrimental effect on the credibility of aromatic oils as medicinal products, an effect which persists today. Beauty therapists tend to focus on the aesthetic effects in aiding wellbeing, using pre-blended oils which are classified simply as 'relaxing', 'stimulating', 'energising' or some other equally nebulous criterion which does not allow for individualised treatments. Spas and salons also often offer for sale a wide range of essential oil-containing beauty products, such as face creams, bath gels or aromatic candles, which, while pleasant, serve only to re-emphasise the wellbeing approach suitable for the general public and detract from aromatherapy as a possible clinical modality.

It has taken most of the 20th century to bring aromatherapy into the fold of healthcare. The aromatherapy profession has now developed into one which encompasses many different aspects, ranging from purely scientific research on individual essential oils to a clinical discipline used both in its own right and as a complement to conventional healthcare. Improvements in education, practice and regulation in complementary medicine have added to this progress, with education being firmly separated from commercial oil production. In clinical aromatherapy practice, an understanding of the biological sciences of chemistry, pharmacology and anatomy and physiology, with related pathology, is vital to the safe use of essential oils. The artistic elements of aromatherapy include the aesthetic blending of the oils, competence in their methods of administration and perhaps an appreciation of the principles of energies with which essential oils are thought to be imbued. It is important not to forget the overall philosophy of aromatherapy: in keeping with other complementary therapies, it is the inter-relationship between body, mind and spirit that makes aromatherapy a holistic therapy.

It is possible to view essential oils simply as another pharmacological agent with which to treat physiological symptoms and pathological conditions, but while there is plenty of research evidence on their metabolism, together with studies on their purported therapeutic properties, there is also an increasing amount of investigation into the psychological effects of the oils.

Contemporary regulation of aromatherapy

In the United Kingdom, regulation of the complementary therapy professions has been through considerable change in the last 20 years or so. Previously, under 16th-century Common Law in England and Wales, anyone could practise any form of healthcare which was not already statutorily regulated. It was therefore unlawful (and still is) to practise as a midwife, doctor, nurse or dentist – only those on the relevant national registers were permitted to practise these professions. However, during the 1980s and 1990s, the growing public interest in complementary medicine led to a number of explorations about the 'professionalisation' of individual therapies. Osteopathy and chiropractic became statutorily regulated in the mid-1990s, with practitioners governed by the General Osteopathic Council or General Chiropractic Council. Several other fields of complementary medicine, notably those which were already well disciplined with prescribed programmes of education and a reasonable or emerging body of research evidence, such as herbal medicine and Western acupuncture, chose voluntary self-regulation. Although there remains no legal requirement for all practitioners of these therapies to become members of the regulatory organisations, those who choose not to do so are considered less credible and often find it difficult to obtain appropriate indemnity insurance cover.

However, there are no laws directly governing aromatherapy practice and there is no obligation on the part of the therapist to be a member of one of the regulatory organisations. There are numerous aromatherapy training institutions and professional registers, the main ones being the International Federation of Professional Aromatherapists (IFPA) and the Aromatherapy Council, which sets itself out to be the lead body for, and the 'voice of', aromatherapy in the United Kingdom. In addition, in 2007, the General Regulatory Council for Complementary Therapists (GRCCT) was set up, and the Complementary and Natural Healthcare Council (CNHC) followed in 2008. These organisations act as voluntary regulators for complementary practitioners of various disciplines, including aromatherapy and massage.

For midwives and doulas using aromatherapy in their care of pregnant and childbearing women, massage and essential oils are seen as additional tools to enhance their practice. It is not a professional requirement to be a fully qualified aromatherapist, but aromatherapy must be used within the parameters of existing training and regulation. Midwives and other maternity professionals must remain cognisant of the fact that they are *not* qualified or employed as aromatherapists and should not undertake any aspect of aromatherapy for which they have not been trained and which is inappropriate for maternity clients. (See Chapter 5 for a detailed discussion on professional accountability.)

EU Directives

In the United Kingdom, herbal medicines, including aromatherapy oils, were previously regulated under sections 12(1) and 12(2) of the Medicines Act 1968. This allowed for exemption from regulation of 'unlicensed herbal remedies', either when made up for individual clients or sold over-the-counter, on condition that the preparation contained only herbal ingredients (except certain prohibited herbs). The EU Medicines Directive 2001 required manufactured herbal preparations to have evidence of safety, effectiveness for specified conditions and a quality assurance system for the manufacturing process. This was replaced in 2004 by the EU Directive, which requires all herbal medicines to have either a full marketing authorisation or a traditional herbal registration. In the United Kingdom the traditional herbal medicines registration scheme is administered by the Medicines and Healthcare Regulatory Authority (MHRA). Registration of a herbal remedy as a medicinal product must demonstrate a history of at least 30 years' use, evidence of safety, adherence to the required manufacturing standards and the provision of appropriate patient information. Many traditional herbal medicines have been granted registration, including St John's wort and black cohosh.

However, aromatherapy falls outside these regulations as essential oils are still considered to be 'cosmetics'. The EU Cosmetics regulations came into force in 2013 and apply to any substance intended for contact with external parts of the human body for the purposes of perfuming, cleaning, protecting them and keeping them in good condition. Since aromatherapists must not, by law, make any medicinal claims for their products, it is deemed that most essential oils used by practitioners fall into this category. Therapists who prepare blends when there has been a one-to-one consultation with the client are thus largely unaffected by the 2004 EU Directive and come under Regulation 3 of the Human Medicines Regulations 2012, which has replaced section 12(1) of the 1968 Medicines Act.

Within maternity care, it is therefore permissible for a midwife or doula to prepare a blend of essential and carrier oils for an individual mother, following a one-to-one consultation, with the first treatment being provided by the practitioner. Any unused oil can then be given to the mother to take home, with a detailed information sheet, and the bottle clearly labelled and intended only for use by the individual mother. The oil blend should generally be prepared at the time of the consultation. If the midwife or doula uses a pre-prepared blend of essential oil, this should be a commercially produced product.

However, in some maternity units, midwives may prepare a blend to use for a specific condition, such as in a 'post-dates pregnancy' clinic. This is acceptable on condition that an individual consultation with each mother is undertaken, although the midwife is not legally allowed to make a claim that the blend will actually facilitate labour onset. Specifying that the blend is for 'natural induction' must be based on the relaxation effects in reducing cortisol and increasing oxytocin release, rather than on the pharmacological properties of each essential oil, as this would constitute a medicinal product for which a licence would be required. The midwife who takes responsibility for blending the oils must be an appropriately trained member of staff (in order to be covered by the hospital's vicarious liability insurance). (See Chapter 5 for more on training.)

Maternity professionals who wish to prepare aromatherapy products for distribution or supply to the community in general, whether for sale or free of charge, are bound by the EU Directives on cosmetics and should also be fully qualified aromatherapists. They will also be bound by the Human Medicines Regulations relating to the sale and supply of medicinal substances and to section 7 on traditional herbal remedies (see www.legislation.gov.uk/uksi/2012).

What are essential oils?

Plant essential oils are produced during the process of photosynthesis and stored in the flowers, leaves, fruit, seeds and other parts of all plants. They are highly volatile, aromatic, fluid constituents usually found in tiny droplets in the veins, glands, glandular hairs and sacs of plants. Their function is to act as regulators, hormones and catalysts, and to assist the plant in adapting to environments that would normally be stressful, thus promoting greater growth. Essential oils act as a protection for the plant against disease, parasites and extremes of temperature – in hot areas, protection from the sun, and in cold areas, protection against frost and snow. The varying aromas of essential oils help to attract specific insects for pollination and some essential oils may act as natural weed-killers in the surrounding soil. They are often coloured and are fat soluble, so they do not dissolve easily in water but mix well with vegetable oils, fats and waxes.

Some plants yield a minute amount of essential oil compared with others. For example, over 2000 kg of rose petals are required to produce just 1 kg of essential oil, making true rose oil extremely expensive. Compare this to the ease with which essential oil of orange can be obtained – most people will have experienced a spurt of liquid into their face when peeling an orange, which is some of the essential oil from the pores in the skin being expressed and not, as might be assumed, just the juice from the fruit.

The chemical constituents of individual essential oils may vary, depending on the geographical terrain, climate, time of day and the season. For example, high-altitude Alpine lavender oil smells much fresher and sweeter than lavender oil obtained from plants grown at lower altitudes. Another example is jasmine: the aroma of jasmine flowers, from which the essential oil is obtained, is much stronger at night; and because the petals are delicate, the flowers must be picked by hand during the hours of darkness, making this another very expensive essential oil. Conversely, rose petals must be picked in the early morning so that any dew is retained.

Different parts of the same plant may yield different essential oils – for example, from the orange tree can be extracted essential oils of orange (from the peel), neroli (from the blossom) and an unusual woody-smelling oil called petitgrain, which comes from the twigs. Many of the essential oils derived from culinary herbs, such as rosemary, sage or marjoram, have been extracted from the leaves, as are oils such as eucalyptus. Others are extracted from the fruit peel (especially the citrus oils such as orange, lemon, bergamot, lime and grapefruit), from the flowers (including neroli, ylang ylang and chamomile), from seeds (carrot seed and black pepper) or from the bark or wood chips from the tree (frankincense, sandalwood and rosewood).

Extraction of essential oils from plants

Aromatherapy is part of the wider discipline of herbal medicine. However, the essential oils used in aromatherapy have a different composition from those used in medical herbalism, because the extraction process used to produce essential oils suitable for use in aromatherapy recovers the smaller, lighter molecules. The method of extraction of the essential oils depends on the part of the plant from which the oil is derived and the difficulty in this process. Most essential oils are fairly readily extracted through a process of steam or water distillation, as with lavender, or by expression, suitable for the citrus oils. Other, more complicated, procedures may be necessary for essential oils from petals, as the delicate flowers would be damaged by simple expression or steam distillation.

The following is a brief summary of the different methods:

- *Steam distillation:* This is the most economical method of extraction and involves the use of water vapour, which is passed over and through the plant material at high pressure. The volatility of the essential oils means that they are forced from the plant cells and are then cooled, condensed and collected; the oil and water then separate out. The water parts of the initial distillation are called hydrosols or floral waters, which are used for skin care and perfume production.

- *Water distillation:* The plant material is immersed in water, heated to boiling point and the steam then carries the essential oils out of the plants. (This can be achieved by hanging a bunch of lavender under the hot water tap of the bath, and the essential oils will pass from the plant material into the bath water). The water protects some constituents from over-heating, but this can be a long process and other constituents can be damaged by the water.

- *Percolation or hydro-diffusion:* This is a newer method of extracting essential oils which is similar to steam distillation but quicker and simpler. Steam percolates downwards through the plant material, and then the essential oil and the steam are condensed, as with steam distillation.

- *Expression:* This method is commonly used to extract essential oils such as lemon, orange, bergamot and tangerine. Pressure is used to squeeze the essential oils out. This was originally performed by hand but is now done via mechanical means.

- *Solvent extraction:* This is generally used for the oils which are more difficult – and thus more expensive – to extract, including rose, jasmine and neroli. The plant material is soaked in organic solvents (e.g. acetone, hexane, methanol or toluene), which cause the oils, and other constituents (e.g. waxes, resins, chlorophyll and pigments) to dissolve out of the plant. The residue is then repeatedly washed to obtain the maximum yield and cooled, when it solidifies into a wax substance. The wax is removed by washing with alcohol, leaving the essential oil, the final residue being called an absolute.

- *Carbon dioxide extraction:* This is a popular but expensive and complicated process which produces oils of very high quality. Liquid carbon dioxide is pressurised to become a 'super critical' substance which is neither a liquid nor a gas, allowing the organic molecules of the essential oils to dissolve, after which the carbon dioxide returns to being a gas.

Purchasing quality essential oils for aromatherapy practice

In clinical aromatherapy, it is vital to use high-quality essential oils to ensure purity. Most of the essential oils produced from plants are used by the food and perfumery industries, with only a small proportion being used for the clinical aromatherapy market. Perhaps the only sure way to obtain the best quality essential oils would be to buy organically produced oils, but there appears to be little evidence to suggest that those essential oils which are produced via organic farming methods result in substances which are any more clinically effective than those which are mass-produced. It is not really necessary to buy organically produced oils for maternity care, given the relatively small amounts which will be used for women during pregnancy, labour or the postnatal period (although aromatherapists working on a daily basis may prefer to do so for their own protection).

In clinical aromatherapy, an essential oil is chosen for its supposed therapeutic properties due to the balance of the known chemical constituents. If, however, a particular batch of essential oil lacks some of those chemical constituents, perhaps due to climatic conditions, the physiological effects on the client receiving treatment with these oils may be different from those anticipated. It is important to maintain a record of the batch number of each new bottle of essential oils, in the same way as one would record the batch number of drugs. This will also help in the event of repeated adverse reactions occurring when using oils from a particular batch, as the oil can then be returned for analysis to the company from which it has been purchased.

Occasionally a supplier may attempt to add chemical constituents which are known to be missing from a particular batch of essential oil, either from another essential oil or a synthetic substance. This is one reason why it is wise to purchase essential oils only from one, or a maximum of two, suppliers whom you come to know well enough to be sure of the quality of the oils. An increasing number of essential oil suppliers will provide, on request, a chromatographic analysis of the oil being purchased, with a guarantee of quality control mechanisms. Even though you may not understand these written analyses, the very fact that they can be provided is sufficient proof of reasonable quality. Chromatography enables analysis of essential oils (and other chemical products) by producing, in effect, a 'fingerprint' of the oils and may be used when the purity of the essential oil is in question. The analysis of the essential oil is matched against the known chemical profile of the specific oil, and shows the presence or absence of undesirable constituents. Box 2.1 provides a summary of the issues relating to the purchase of essential oils.

Box 2.1 Purchasing essential oils for clinical aromatherapy

Purchase from a reputable supplier who
produces essential oils for clinical use.

Use only one, or a maximum of two suppliers, and get to know them.

Suppliers should be able, on request, to produce
evidence of purity and lack of contamination.

Essential oils should be packaged in small, dark,
glass bottles with a dropper in the neck.

Packaging should include safety data, expiry date and a batch number.

Purchase small bottles to avoid oxidisation
of unused oils in larger bottles.

Storage of essential oils

Essential oils are expensive and should be stored in a way that will preserve their chemical properties for as long as possible. Physically, essential oils deteriorate (oxidise) when exposed to oxygen, light, changing temperatures or other chemicals (see Chapter 3). When purchasing the oils, they should be in dark bottles, usually brown, green or blue; essential oils displayed in beautifully crafted clear glass bottles may look lovely and smell normal at the time of purchase, but they will deteriorate quickly and are not suitable for clinical aromatherapy. The pure essential oils should also be in glass bottles, since synthetic plastic will expedite the process of oxidisation. Whilst it is acceptable to blend essential oils with carrier oil into a plastic container for immediate use, they should never be stored in plastic.

Oxygen also triggers oxidisation – every time a bottle is opened, oxygen will enter and mix with the essential oil. It is therefore wise to purchase oils in small quantities. Most essential oils can be bought in 10 ml bottles, which gives 200 drops, or possibly up to 100 treatments. Larger bottles will take longer for the oil to be used up, with a consequently longer period of time for deterioration to occur. Further, when choosing a selection of essential oils for clinical use, it is better to have a small selection of different oils which offer versatility rather than a large number of oils, some of which may hardly ever be used.

Some essential oils, particularly the citrus oils, should be kept out of the sun and in a cool dark place to avoid rapid deterioration. In an institutional setting it would be better to keep the full selection of essential oils in one place, such as a small drugs refrigerator, which legally must be lockable for security purposes. Although most essential oils maintain their properties for up to a year, citrus oils, even when stored in the refrigerator, will keep for only 3–6 months after opening. Storing oils other than the citrus oils in the refrigerator will not damage them; occasionally, some oils may solidify slightly in the cold, but this can be reversed simply by holding the bottle in the palm of the hand to warm it. If, at any time, a bottle is opened and the aroma is different from that expected, especially when compared to other bottles of the same essential oil, the open bottle should be discarded as oxidisation is likely to have occurred, causing the chemical constituents to alter.

Essential oils should be kept unblended for as long as possible because once they are mixed with a carrier oil or another essential oil, the oxidisation process will commence. If oils which are pre-blended by the midwife or doula are deemed necessary to practice, they must be adequately labelled with the essential and carrier oils used and the percentage of the blend. They must also have a 'use by' date of no more than four weeks from the date of blending, to avoid administration of blends in which the chemical structure may have been altered through oxidisation.

Blending of oils for individual women at the time of a treatment allows for increased maternal choice and more autonomy for the caregiver, as well as less risk of wastage from pre-blended oils. There are some exceptions, when the choice of suitable essential oils is limited – for example, if midwives offer a clinic for women who are past their estimated due dates, there may be a standard blend of essential oils used for the treatment. This means that the oils can be pre-blended on-site and used for this specific group of women, subject to adherence to the expiry date and storage requirements, as well as the EU legalities.

When essential oils are added to water, which consists of the chemicals hydrogen and oxygen, the process of oxidisation will commence immediately. If essential oils are blended in water, perhaps for a facial spray to refresh a woman in labour, this mix will only last for 24 hours and should then be discarded. There is, of course, no real problem if essential oils are added to the bath, as women will only spend a short period of time in the water. Box 2.2 summarises the requirements for the safe and appropriate storage of essential oils.

Box 2.2 Storage of essential oils

Essential oils should remain unopened until needed.

Only open one bottle of each essential oil at any one time.

Be aware of 'use by' dates for the different essential oils.

Citrus, and some other oils, should be stored in the refrigerator.

In institutional settings it is wise to store all essential oils in a single locked refrigerator.

Discard any oils if the aroma is different from that expected.

Blend oils only as needed.

Store blended oils in dark glass bottles, with a 'use by' date of no more than four weeks.

Essential oils added to water last a maximum of 24 hours.

Blended oils must be labelled with the specific essential oils and carrier oil, percentage blend, named user (if appropriate), expiry date and safety data.

Oils blended for a named mother should also be labelled with her name.

Dosages in maternity aromatherapy

In aromatherapy practice, the normal maximum dose of an essential oil blend for massage would be 3% for a fit, healthy, non-pregnant adult. The dose would be adjusted for children, the elderly or for people with a medical condition. In pregnancy the dose will normally be 1% and should not exceed 1.5%; in labour this can be increased, with 2% being used for any treatments provided during labour and for the duration of the puerperium, up to at least eight weeks postpartum. Once the mother's body has returned to the non-pregnant state, she can be given the normal adult 3% dose. There is also one exception during late pregnancy: 3% can be used when blending oils for women with a post-dates pregnancy. Ideally, the practitioner should use the minimum amount of essential oil required to produce a therapeutic effect, but this will depend on how many essential oils are used and how much carrier oil is needed. (See also Chapter 4 for information on over-dosing.)

To calculate a dose for massage, it is necessary first to decide how much carrier oil is needed, depending on the type of treatment. For example, a foot or hand massage will require no more than 5 ml of carrier oil, a back massage will require around 10 ml and a full body massage will require up to 25 ml or even 30 ml, according to the mother's size. The amount of carrier oil needed can also be affected by the skin – women with very dry skin will need more as they will absorb it more quickly than women with normal or oily skin.

To each 5 ml of carrier oil should then be added the required number of drops of essential oil. For a 1% blend, this is just a single drop of essential oil; for a 2% blend, 2 drops would be added; and for a 3% blend, 3 drops would be added.

Thus for a 2% blend, using three essential oils in 25 ml of carrier oil, the calculation would be:

- 25 ml of carrier oil = 5 x 5 ml
- 2% = 2 drops per 5 ml = 10 drops of essential oil.

For a quick reference guide to dosages for massage, see Table 2.1. For dosages for the bath, compresses, etc. see page 56.

Table 2.1 Dosages used in massage

MAXIMUM PERCENTAGE BLEND PERMITTED	PRECONCEPTION AND PREGNANCY	LABOUR AND POSTNATAL	POST-DATES PREGNANCY 'NATURAL INDUCTION' ONLY
	1–1.5%	2%	3%

PERCENTAGE BLEND REQUIRED	NUMBER OF DROPS TO BE ADDED PER:			
	5 ML CARRIER OIL	10 ML CARRIER OIL	15 ML CARRIER OIL	20 ML CARRIER OIL
1%	1	2	3	4
1.5%	N/A	3	N/A	6
2%	2	4	6	8
3%	3	6	9	12

Source: Tiran 2014

Blending of essential oils

Blending is part of the creative, artistic side of aromatherapy. Several essential oils can be blended together for their therapeutic characteristics, but the aroma must also be aesthetically pleasing to the mother. The choice of specific essential oils will depend on several factors, including the purpose of the proposed treatment and any relevant contraindications or precautions according to the mother's clinical condition.

In general aromatherapy, many authorities will use up to five different essential oils in a blend, but in maternity care it is wise to limit blending to three oils in total. In the event of side-effects developing, this will enable a more rapid identification of which essential oil may be to blame. Whilst it is sometimes appropriate to use a single essential oil in a carrier oil, this is not normally recommended, for two reasons. First, a synergistic or enhanced effect is achieved by using several essential oils together. This can help to even out the balance of the aromas, particularly if one essential oil has a strong aroma. It can also balance the therapeutic effects – for example, an essential oil which has a sedative effect can be countered by adding a stimulating essential oil to the blend. Second, when intending to administer the oils via a massage, there may be limitations on the recommended percentage blend of certain essential oils which carry a risk of adverse skin reactions, such as bergamot, clary sage, lavender and jasmine (Tisserand and Young 2014). Using these oils in combination with others will allow for an appropriate percentage blend to be used for the treatment but will, in effect, dilute the proportion of the 'offending' oil (see Chapter 4).

The total number of drops in the blend must not exceed that required when only a single essential oil is used. If, for example, a 2% blend of lavender and mandarin is required, with only 5 ml of carrier oil, this would mean that just 1 drop of each essential oil is added to the carrier oil. However, if more carrier oil is to be used, perhaps for a back massage, the balance of the two essential oils does not have to be equal; it can now be adjusted to produce an aesthetically pleasing aroma. In this example, 10 ml of carrier oil would require 4 drops of essential oil, but the mother may prefer more of the mandarin than the lavender (e.g. 3 drops of mandarin and 1 drop of lavender).

For a full body massage using a 1.5% blend in 30 ml of carrier oil with essential oils of black pepper, lavender and grapefruit, the total number of essential oil drops would be 9 (3 drops per 10 ml). As black pepper has a very distinctive and strong aroma, only 1 drop, or perhaps a maximum of 2 drops, would be used. Conversely, grapefruit (or bergamot) has a much more subtle aroma so a greater number of drops would be needed. The final blend might then be 1 drop of black pepper, 3 drops of lavender and 5 drops of grapefruit. It is wise to be cautious when dispensing drops to ensure the correct number is added to the blend, as some oils have a very thin consistency and will pour readily from the bottle, whereas others may have a thicker consistency, making them slower to dispense.

There are several different methods of choosing which essential oils combine well together to produce a pleasant aroma (see Table 2.2). In perfumery, the 'notes' system of blending is used, developed by the perfumer, Septimum Piesse, in the 19th century, to facilitate the creation of harmonious scents. As a general rule, essential oils extracted from the top parts of plants – the flowers and fruit – are the 'top' notes, providing fresh, fruity aromas immediately noticeable on blending, but which are relatively short-lived. These include the citrus essences and other sharp, distinctive aromas such as eucalyptus. Essential oils from the whole plants, leaves and stems (i.e. the middle part of the plant) constitute the 'middle' notes, which are often used as the main therapeutic oil for the blend. In general aromatherapy, this would include most of the herbal oils such as rosemary, sage and thyme, although these oils are not used in maternity care. The 'base' notes are those essential oils extracted from the base of the plant – for example, the roots, seeds, bark and wood. The true aromas of these 'base' notes emerge only after warming, such as during massage into the skin, but linger the longest. A useful comparison to help understand this concept is to consider the drug Syntometrine, given intramuscularly to aid placental separation. Within this drug, the oxytocin component works rapidly to initiate an almost immediate uterine contraction and to force the placenta to separate from the uterine wall, but its action is short-lived. The work of this 'synergistic' blend of drugs is then taken over by the ergometrine, which takes several minutes to have an effect, but whose action is then sustained to prevent uterine relaxation and consequent haemorrhage.

However, whilst many aromatherapists use the 'notes' system of blending, it is not essential to use this method. Essential oils derived from the same part of different plants will generally blend well – for example, fruit oils, flower oils or herb oils. Essential oils from the same plant family will also blend well together (see Chapter 7), as will those that contain the same chemical constituents, such as the citronella-rich oils, eucalyptus, mandarin and tangerine. A few essential oils, such as lavender and rose, are extremely versatile and blend well with a large number of other oils, whereas others with a very distinctive aroma, including tea tree, may have limited flexibility.

Table 2.2 Aromas of some chemical constituents found in essential oils

CHEMICAL CONSTITUENT	AROMA	ESSENTIAL OIL
Aldehydes		
Citral	Citrus, lemon	Mandarin/tangerine
Citronellal	Citrus, rose	Lemon
Esters		
Benzyl acetate	Floral, fruity	Ylang ylang
Linalyl acetate	Light, herbal, slightly fruity	Clary sage
Neryl acetate	Sweet, rose-like, fruity	Neroli
Alcohols		
Cedrol	Faintly woody	Cypress
Citronellol	Rich, floral, rose-like	Geranium
Menthol	Fresh, minty	Peppermint
Nerol	Sweet, floral, slightly sea-weedy	Neroli
Monoterpenes		
Limonene	Weak citrus	Grapefruit
Myrcene	Sweet, balsamic	Black pepper
Phellandrene	Citrus, spicy, woody	Frankincense
Sesquiterpenes		
α-terpinene	Fresh, citrus	Tea tree
β-bisabolene	Balsamic, spicy	Chamomile

In fairness, much of the art of blending of essential oils comes from an instinctive feel for what is right, and some practitioners are better at blending than others. The first priority is to choose at least one essential oil which is intended to achieve the required therapeutic response – for example, a relaxing oil, a stimulating oil, an analgesic oil or a strongly anti-infective oil. It may be that two or even all three of the essential oils chosen for an individual mother will have the same effects – a wonderfully relaxing blend might be lavender and ylang ylang, which are both relaxing, with a lighter citrus oil to lighten the overall aroma. Although citrus oils are not directly relaxing, they enhance the mood and, in maternity aromatherapy, are the 'fall back' oils of choice – if in doubt about how to produce a pleasant blend, use at least one of the citrus oils (bergamot, grapefruit, lemon, lime, mandarin/ tangerine, neroli, petitgrain, sweet orange, etc.).

Blending should be a partnership between the practitioner and the mother. When helping a mother to choose an appropriate blend for her treatment, the practitioner should identify one or two oils which will have the desired therapeutic effect. This can be discussed with the mother, trying to elicit what types of aromas she enjoys. It can be useful to ask her what type of perfume she likes – light and fruity, heavy and sensual or spicy and masculine. The mother (and the midwife) should not smell *all* the oils being considered as appropriate to the treatment. Following discussion with the mother, the practitioner can make some suggestions, based on knowledge and experience, and then identify the three essential oils which best suit the situation. The mother can then be invited to smell the chosen blend to see if it is to her liking. This can be done by removing the bottle tops of the selected essential oils, holding the open bottles together and passing them under the mother's nose, although she should not allow her face to come into contact with the bottle tops. The mother should breathe normally and be discouraged from taking a deep breath. If the mother likes the blend in principle but finds one essential oil rather strong, the practitioner can lower the relevant bottle and let her smell the oils again. If she is still unsure, another essential oil can be suggested to replace the one which she dislikes. (Alternatively, special tapers can be bought, similar to those used in perfumery stores: a single drop of essential oil is put on the end and the mother can then smell it, although this is rather wasteful in maternity settings.) On no account should either the mother or the practitioner smell numerous different oils, either singly or in combination, as the nostrils will become saturated with the molecules from those oils inhaled first, making it difficult to elicit the aromas of those smelled later.

Many essential oils work synergistically together; in other words, essential oils achieve a greater effectiveness when blended with others than if used individually and separately. Each essential oil will have many different therapeutic actions, some of which will be useful in specific circumstances. The principle of synergy also extends to the individual chemical constituents, with the effects of a whole essential oil being greater than if the individual components were used in isolation. An example of this is seen in the case of lavender oil, which has a sedative action greater than the sedative effects of two of its principal constituents, linalyl acetate and linalool (Adorjan and Buchbauer 2010). Other chemical constituents have an antagonistic effect, such as in rosemary, which contains spasmolytic 1.8 cineole as well as α-pinene, which has the opposite effect. When combining essential oils with the intention of achieving a specific clinical effect, it is possible to use oils which have opposing actions yet which will have a more positive result than if a single oil was used. For example, Hongratanaworakit (2011) demonstrated a greater reduction in anxiety when using lavender combined with bergamot, than in a placebo control group.

Although blending is an art which can take considerable experience to do well, there are some simple guidelines which may help the novice (see Box 2.3). This will give an idea of whether or not the essential oils enhance or compete with one another, but it is only with continued practice that individuals become 'tuned in' and adept at selecting oils that blend well. In Chapter 7, each essential oil has been chosen as blending well with most of the others in the selection provided.

Box 2.3 Principles for blending of essential oils

Determine the therapeutic effect required from the treatment.

Choose one essential oil which is notable for this effect.

Choose one or two other essential oils to make an aroma which is aesthetically pleasing to both the mother and the person giving the treatment – these may have similar therapeutic effects or different effects.

Do not use any essential oils if the mother dislikes the aroma.

In maternity aromatherapy, use no more than three essential oils in a blend.

Decide how much carrier oil is required for the treatment and, from this, calculate the total number of drops of essential oil.

Now decide on the proportion of each essential oil. (NB The more carrier oil that is used, the greater the number of essential oil drops that can be used, allowing for increased flexibility in deciding the proportions of each individual essential oil.)

Methods of administration of essential oils

Essential oils can be administered in many different ways. Dermal administration methods include massage, compresses, baths and footbaths. Direct administration to the respiratory tract is via inhalation in a vaporiser or on a tissue or taper. The method of administration often contributes to the overall effectiveness of the treatment – especially massage – although the method selected may depend on several factors. The condition to be treated may dictate this – for example, a cough or cold is best treated by inhalation to enable the essential oils to act directly on the respiratory tract. Conversely, women wanting aromatherapy in pregnancy for relaxation could perhaps benefit most from having a massage.

Time may play a part too. Midwives using aromatherapy in their clinical practice may have time constraints brought about by staffing levels and workload. Adding essential oils to the bath or a foot bath, or offering a short foot or hand massage may result in a more equitable service for the women in their care. Caring for labouring women is normally in a one-to-one situation when there may be more time for massage, but the mother's condition may influence the method of administration, such as her request for intermittent treatment between contractions. On the other hand, incorporating aromatherapy massage into midwifery practice may allow more time to sit and talk with the woman.

The mother's preference for a particular method must be taken into account. Some women dislike being touched, especially in labour, and this must be respected by offering alternative ways of receiving the benefits of essential oils. For example, some women will prefer showering to bathing so adding essential oils to the bath water may not be realistic.

Administration of essential oils via the respiratory tract: inhalation

Inhalation of essential oils occurs with *all* methods of administration: if the aroma is noticeable in the air, everyone in the room will be inhaling the essential oil molecules, which will then pass down the respiratory tract to the lungs and throughout the circulation. (See Chapter 3 on physiology and Chapter 4 on safety.)

There are many items of equipment now available to facilitate diffusion of the essential oils into the atmosphere. Some are decorative pots which incorporate a small night-light-type candle, the heat of the flame helping to evaporate the volatile essential oils. Any equipment involving a naked flame is not, however, appropriate for use within an institutional setting because of fire regulations, and extreme care should be taken if a mother wishes to use one at home. She should be advised about safe positioning of the vaporiser, remembering that, in labour, she may inadvertently move an arm or leg which could knock it over. Electrical vaporisers are also available, but if a mother wishes to bring one of these into the maternity unit for use during labour, safety of the electrical wiring must be checked in advance. There are several types of electrical diffusers, including: 'aroma stones', which produce mild heat to warm the volatile essential oils; aroma-lamps, which use water to warm the oils; mist diffusers for facial or room sprays; nebulisers, which are generally used for respiratory conditions.

Many people like to use these vaporisers to provide a pleasant aroma within the room. However, it is the opinion of this author that the use of vaporisers within a maternity unit, midwife-led birth centre or other institutional setting is inappropriate, unethical and sometimes dangerous. At the very least, some individuals exposed to the volatile oils may dislike the aromas. Most importantly, administration of the chemicals within the oils could have deleterious effects on the mother, fetus, relatives or staff (see Chapter 4). Mothers may wish to use vaporisers in their own homes but should be advised not to use them for more than 10–15 minutes at a time, to avoid overpowering the nostrils with essential oil molecules, which can lead to headaches, nausea and drowsiness.

There are, however, some situations in which inhalation as a direct method of administering essential oils can be very useful. It is a logical means of treating conditions specifically affecting the respiratory tract, such as colds, influenza and sinus congestion, or post-operative chest infections. It can also be useful as a focused inhalation aimed at providing an immediate effect, although generally this is not long lasting. For example, waves of nausea in labour can be reduced if the mother is able to inhale an appropriate essential oil with an anti-emetic effect (e.g. peppermint) but this would not be a suitable method of administration for a woman experiencing ongoing sickness in pregnancy (see Chapter 3). Acute situations such as panic in labour may respond well to inhalation of an oil such as frankincense, but again chronic stress during pregnancy is best treated with a method of administration which will prolong the effects of the oils. Essential oils can be administered on a cotton wool ball, gauze swab, tissue or via a taper (such as those used in perfumery departments and also available from essential oil suppliers). A single drop can be added and the mother can then inhale it directly as needed. The swab, tissue, taper, etc. should be discarded after two hours and a fresh one used if required (see Chapter 3).

In oncology care, Stringer and Donald (2011) used Aromasticks®, a relatively new means of respiratory administration, to empower patients to manage their own symptoms of anxiety, sleep disturbance and nausea. These are similar to commercially available nasal sticks for congestion (e.g. Vicks®), but are provided blank so that essential oils can be added as appropriate. A more recent study by Schneider (2015) on the use of Aromasticks® in the treatment of stress demonstrated reduced heart rate, blood pressure and cortisol levels. Aromasticks® have not yet been formally used in maternity care and warrant further investigation before being implemented as a method of administering essential oils, although the initial studies look promising. Midwives and others working with pregnant and labouring women would need to be very clear about the way in which these sticks are used and should not see them as a panacea for everything, nor as merely a fragrance inhaler. The chemistry of the essential oils, particularly the rate of deterioration, needs to be taken into account and clear, evidence-based information should be available to women if these are to be used. In addition, the EU regulations need to be adhered to in terms of individual consultations.

Administration of essential oils via the skin: massage

Within midwifery, massage and touch have always been an integral part of the care of childbearing women. Even today, many cultures around the world incorporate massage and herbal remedies into labour care, including back and abdominal massage for labour pain and perineal massage to ease the passage of the fetal head. Nurturing touch, as opposed to functional touch, can be a profound experience, especially during labour. Spencer (2004) considers that compassionate touch is virtually non-existent within the medical model of maternity care, with touch being used primarily as a diagnostic tool or as a manipulative technique, or even, perhaps, as a method of restraint. She debates the types of touch employed by traditional midwives and birth doulas, focusing on: comforting touch as a means of pain relief; therapeutic and healing touch, in which various strategies (e.g. pressure point work) are used to aid progress; 'greeting touch', in which the infant is gently placed in contact with the mother's body; 'blessing touch', which 'supports the social and spiritual orientation of the mother'.

Touch can have direct psychological effects, and caution should be taken with women who have a history of abuse (domestic or sexual). Some women dislike certain parts of their body being touched, such as the abdomen, breasts or inner thighs, although they may accept a massage which does not involve these areas. Cultural aspects may also play a part in a woman's receptiveness to massage and touch. Asian women, for example, are brought up with massage being used regularly in many families, whereas women from Western countries may be more reticent, although it is wise to refrain from making too many generalisations.

In some countries, inhalation is the preferred method of administration of essential oils, but the link between aromatherapy and the beauty therapy industry in Britain has perpetuated the use of massage as the principal way of applying them. The application of an essential oil blend via the skin is certainly enhanced when given via massage, and most women will report that massage is the most relaxing and enjoyable method of receiving the benefits of the aromatic oils. In itself, massage can be mentally and physically relaxing whilst also being revitalising. Massage is a combination of touch, pressure and vibration which helps to stimulate the circulatory and excretory processes (urinary, intestinal, lymphatic and integumentary). It relaxes and tones muscles and assists the woman, quite literally, to get 'in touch' – physically and emotionally – with herself.

There are many different types of massage, which are often used in conjunction with one another. Each type involves different techniques, pressures and vibrational movements. The commonest types used in aromatherapy involve a combination of Swedish soft-tissue massage and deeper lymphatic and neuro-muscular massage. Occasionally, other forms of touch therapy will be integrated into the treatment, such as reflexology, shiatsu, acupressure or reiki (Therapeutic Touch or spiritual healing). However, it is not the purpose of this book to cover these therapies, which are distinctly different from the touch therapy used for the administration of essential oils (see Tiran 2010b; Yates 2003). In addition, this book cannot teach the practitioner *how* to perform massage. Basic principles are discussed here and some suggestions for the application of various manual techniques to maternity care are given, but it is left to the practitioner to pursue the acquisition of specific massage skills. Massage is, in any case, mostly intuitive and cannot be learned from a book. There are many excellent courses and more detailed textbooks available elsewhere (see the Resources section and Yates 2010).

Soft-tissue massage consists of several types of movement of the hands:

- *Effleurage* is a slow, flowing movement in which the body part is stroked by the whole hand, which changes to fit the contours of the body. Movements are normally directed towards the heart to stimulate circulation and lymphatic drainage, although effleurage at the end of a massage tends to encourage removal of tension from the body by outwards movement along the limbs and up the face and head. Effleurage may be fairly light (although not so light as to be ticklish), or deeper for work on specific tense muscles and to improve blood flow. Effleurage is used to link other massage movements and can be performed on any part of the body. It is relaxing and enhances a sense of wellbeing. Different pressures and speeds, pausing and holding occasionally, will provide variety in the massage.

- *Petrissage* involves deeper work with the thumbs and fingers on more focused areas of the body. Soft tissues, notably muscles, are compressed either against underlying bone or against themselves, and the movements may be in the form of kneading, wringing, rolling or shaking manipulations.

- *Kneading* is a circular squeezing movement, using the fingers and thumbs to pick up fleshy parts of the body or to compress the tissues against underlying structures. It is a useful technique for dealing with aching and tense muscles as it stimulates local circulation and disperses any lactic acid which may have accumulated in the muscles.

- *Percussion* movements (*tapotement*) include cupping and hacking, perhaps the two movements most readily associated with Swedish massage. They involve brisk bouncy movements on fleshy parts of the body to improve circulation and re-energise the client. Both these techniques should be followed by effleurage to soothe and calm. The movements may be omitted altogether as they can disturb deep relaxation.

There is research evidence to show that moderate-pressure massage enhances immune functioning (Field 2014) and lowers the stress hormone, cortisol (Field *et al.* 2005; Morhenn, Beavin and Zak 2012; Wu *et al.* 2014). It is postulated that the mechanism of action is due to a direct effect on those parts of the brain involved in stress and the regulation of emotions, namely the hypothalamus, amygdala and the anterior cingulate cortex (Field 2014). Other authorities have found a reduction in blood pressure (Liao *et al.* 2014; Mohebbi *et al.* 2014; Nelson 2015) and beneficial effects on the immune system, with increased oxytocin (Major *et al.* 2015). There appears to be an accumulative effect of repeated massages (Rapaport, Schettler and Bresee 2012), although Törnhage *et al.* (2013) found no long-term cortisol reduction with successive treatments, suggesting perhaps that a level of resistance is attained.

Massage has been found to reduce pain post-operatively (Boitor *et al.* 2015), in dysmenorrhoea (Bakhtshirin *et al.* 2015; Marzouk, El-Nemer and Baraka 2013) and in labour (Janssen *et al.* 2012; McNabb *et al.* 2006). Receiving massage antenatally appears to reduce the risk of prematurity and low birth weight, and to alleviate postnatal depression (Field *et al.* 2009; Field *et al.* 2004). Intrapartum massage may increase the duration of breastfeeding (Adams *et al.* 2015), possibly due to an increase in oxytocin (Major *et al.* 2015). During the puerperium, massage can ease anxiety, reduce depression and aid development of the mother–infant relationship (Imura, Misao and Ushijima 2006). Encouraging mothers to perform baby massage may also positively affect maternal mood and cortisol levels (Fujita *et al.* 2006). Table 2.3 outlines the benefits of massage in maternity care. For contraindications and precautions, see Chapter 4.

Table 2.3 Benefits of massage in pregnancy, labour and the puerperium

PHYSICAL	PSYCHOLOGICAL
Relaxes muscles	Mental relaxation
Lowers blood pressure	Reduces stress
Stimulates circulation	Revitalising
Reduces pain	Aids emotional release
Reduces oedema	Facilitates communication
Increases excretion – diuresis, defecation	Aids sleep
Aids lymphatic drainage	Provides time for oneself
Facilitates normal birth, reduces intervention	Increases maternal satisfaction

Administration of essential oils via the skin: in water

Essential oils can be administered in water, such as in the bath or a foot bath, or applied locally as a compress. Contact with the skin causes the oils to absorb down the hair shafts into the circulation. In addition, the heat of the water and the steam encourages greater absorption via the respiratory tract, making baths or foot baths an especially beneficial means of administering the oils.

Essential oils should not be added to the water neat – although they are not actually oily in consistency, they do float on the surface of the water. If the woman came into contact with the oils as she immersed herself in the bath water, she would have neat essential oil on her skin, which could cause contact dermatitis, if susceptible. The 'dose' for essential oils in water is not calculated in percentages as with massage blends. Between 4 and 6 drops of essential oil in total (maximum three oils) can be added, preferably as the water is running into the bath so that the agitation will facilitate the spread of the essential oils throughout the water. For a bath, the neat essential oils should be mixed into a few millilitres of carrier oil (e.g. grapeseed oil). Milk can also be used but it must be full-fat (not semi-skimmed or skimmed) as the essential oils are dispersed through the fatty globules. If a foot bath is to be given, a large bowl is filled with water (hot to touch or cold as required) and 2–3 drops of essential oil can be added. A carrier oil is not necessary in this case, as the oils can be dispersed by hand in this smaller amount of water.

Compresses can be made by soaking a cloth (face flannel, tea towel, etc.) in water to which essential oils have been added. The temperature of the water can be hand-hot or cold, depending on the condition to be treated and the mother's preference. The amount of water will depend on the size of the area to be covered. To each litre of water, 2–3 drops of essential oil can be added, without a carrier oil, and dispersed by hand. The cloth is soaked, excess water is squeezed out so that it is not dripping and the compress is applied to the affected area. The compress may need to be changed regularly, especially if the water is hot as it will cool quickly in the air. This method is good for targeting specific small areas of the body – for example, for a headache, lumbosacral pain in labour, shoulder and neck pain, acute antenatal suprapubic discomfort or oedema of the legs and ankles. For some women, it is also preferable to receiving a massage and enables them to enjoy the benefits of aromatherapy without needing to be touched. Compresses are not, however, the most appropriate method of administration for longer-term problems such as ongoing backache.

Essential oils can also be used in water as a vulval wash, for the treatment of infections, leucorrhoea or for general hygiene and freshening after the birth and to aid perineal healing. To a litre of warm or cool water, 2–3 drops of essential oil can be added without carrier oil. With the mother sitting on a bedpan or over a toilet or bidet, the water is then gently sluiced over the vulval and perineal area. The area should be dried gently and thoroughly afterwards, especially if the purpose of the wash is to aid perineal healing. *Please note: Essential oils should not be added to the birthing pool at all. They should not be added to the bath once the membranes have ruptured, otherwise the mother will need to get out for the bath to be emptied and refilled with clean water. If a woman has received a massage prior to entering the birthing pool there is little risk to the baby, as the oils will have absorbed into the skin or evaporated. Further, whilst essential oils can be added to jacuzzis and saunas, use of these methods is contraindicated in pregnancy, due to the risks of high temperatures and the theoretical risk of amniotic embolism.*

Box 2.4 lists the methods of administration of essential oils suitable for use in midwifery/maternity care and Box 2.5 summarises the principles of administration of essential oils in pregnancy, labour and the puerperium. (See also Chapter 6 for further discussion and justification.)

Box 2.4 Summary of methods of administration of essential oils

Massage: For foot, hand, neck and shoulders, back and full body massage, blend the essential oils in a suitable carrier oil to the correct dosage.

In the bath: Add 4–6 drops of essential oil in approximately 2 ml of carrier oil as the water is running into the bath.

In a foot bath: Add 3–4 drops of essential oil to a bowl of warm or cool water, as preferred, and mix thoroughly.

Compress: Add 3–4 drops of essential oil to 0.5 litres of warm or cool water, then soak a cloth in the water and apply to the relevant body part. (NB Should not to be used for perineal healing.)

Neat: Add a single drop of oil (e.g. frankincense) to the centre of the mother's palm for her to inhale. (NB Essential oils should not normally be applied neat.)

On a tissue, gauze swab or cotton wool ball: Add a maximum of 2 drops of essential oil for the mother to inhale. (NB Only for immediate use, discard after use.)

As a facial spray: Add 2–3 drops of mild essential oil (e.g. grapefruit, bergamot) to boiled, cooled water, for use in labour. (NB Keep in refrigerator and discard after 24 hours.)

Vulval wash: Add 2–3 drops of essential oil to a litre of warm or cool water.

Vaporisation: This is contraindicated in an institutional setting. Mothers wishing to vaporise oils at home should be advised to use an electrical vaporiser (rather than a naked flame) for no longer than 15 minutes at a time.

Box 2.5 Principles of administration of aromatherapy in pregnancy and childbirth

A maximum of three essential oils should be used in a blend.

Dosages: 1–1.5% in pregnancy (i.e. 1 drop of essential oil to 5 ml carrier oil).

Dosages: 2% in labour and during the puerperium (i.e. 2 drops of essential oil to 5 ml carrier oil).

Dosages: 3% for natural induction in post-dates pregnancy only (i.e. 3 drops of essential oil to 5 ml carrier oil).

Ensure that the treatment can be carried out in a safe and private environment.

Obtain verbal informed consent and document it.

Assess skin condition for dryness, sensitivity, etc.

Discuss the choice of oils and the reason for treatment with the mother.

Avoid hypotensive essential oils (e.g. lavender, ylang ylang) in labour if an epidural is *in situ*.

Avoid essential oils which facilitate uterine action (e.g. clary sage, jasmine) when syntocinon is commenced or within one hour of other means of stimulating contractions.

Do not add essential oils directly to the water in the birthing pool.

Do not add essential oils to the water if the mother is labouring in the bath with ruptured membranes.

Avoid abdominal massage if the woman has an anteriorly situated placenta or following a Caesarean section.

Avoid clary sage if the mother has excessive lochia or retained products of conception.

Avoid sedating essential oils (e.g. chamomile, ylang ylang) if the mother has a history of postnatal depression.

Ask the mother to wash her breasts after aromatherapy treatment, prior to putting her baby to the breast.

Chapter 3

The Science of Aromatherapy

This chapter includes discussion on:

- aromatherapy and the skin
- administration of essential oils via inhalation
- chemistry of essential oils
- pharmacokinetics of essential oils
- concept of energy in aromatherapy
- difficulties of producing an evidence base for aromatherapy
- evidence of the therapeutic effects of aromatherapy
- evidence in relation to maternity aromatherapy.

Introduction

This chapter deals with the scientific basis of aromatherapy. It is important for midwives and other professionals using essential oils in their care of pregnant, labouring and newly birthed mothers to have an understanding of the anatomy, physiology and chemistry involved in clinical aromatherapy in order to justify and defend its use, particularly with a client group which is vulnerable insofar as physio-psychological wellbeing is compromised, even when pregnancy is progressing normally. It is especially imperative to be able to justify the use of essential oils at this time, since aromatherapy is often denigrated as simply being nice-smelling oils and massage, with any effects being attributed to relaxation and/or the placebo effect. Professionals working with maternity clients must also appreciate that aromatherapy is a clinical modality with many benefits, but also with certain risks when used inappropriately. In addition, it is a holistic therapy aimed at improving wellbeing. As we know, part of the impact of aromatherapy derives from the physiological effects, whilst the nurturing aspects of treatment can have a deeper psychological and spiritual effect. To this end, the concept of energy is also discussed briefly in this chapter. Finally, an improved awareness of the evidence which supports aromatherapy will assist maternity workers to defend their practice and will contribute towards improved practice with enhanced therapeutic effects.

Aromatherapy and the skin

In the United Kingdom, the most commonly used method of administration of essential oils is via the skin, either as a massage or in water (bath, compress, etc.) (see Chapter 2). The skin is the largest organ in the body, occupying over two square metres, and is the primary component of the integumentary system, together with accessory structures such as the hair, nails, sebaceous and sweat glands. Some areas of the body, such as the palms and soles, are covered with very thick skin, whereas others, such as the eyelids, have a very thin covering. Skin acts as a protective cover for the internal organs and prevents body fluids from being lost and harmful substances such as micro-organisms from gaining entry. It is virtually waterproof but allows the passage of certain molecules, including essential oils, as well as harmful soluble chemicals. When the body is warm, temperature control is achieved through the excretion of sweat, which cools on exposure to the air, as well as by vasodilatation and heat radiation. In cool temperatures vasoconstriction acts as an insulating mechanism to enable the body to retain heat. Excretion of some waste materials, such as urea and nitrogen, occurs via the skin. Useful ultraviolet rays convert 7-dehydrocholesterol into vitamin D, while harmful ultraviolet light is screened out by healthy skin.

The outer layer of the skin, the epidermis, is composed of stratified squamous epithelial tissue. It has no blood vessels, but as it is very thin, most cuts and abrasions penetrate the dermal layer beneath and therefore draw blood. Within the epidermis there are between three and five layers depending on the thickness of the skin, starting with the stratum corneum, which consists of parallel rows of dead cells of soft keratin to maintain the skin's elasticity and to protect the living cells beneath from drying out due to exposure to the air. The dead cells are constantly being shed and replaced by cells pushed up from the germinative layer below. The soles of the feet and the palms of the hands also contain the stratum lucidum layer, made up of dead skin cells, which acts as an ultraviolet filter to protect from sunburn, and the stratum granulosum containing keratohyaline granules needed for the process of keratinisation. The next layer is the stratum spinosum, which serves as a support and binding and facilitates the process of protein synthesis leading to cell division and growth. Finally, the stratum basale divides the epidermis from the dermis and helps to produce new cells to replace those lost at the surface. Within the epidermis there are also Langerhans cells, which enhance the body's immune system through phagocytosis and which help activate other white blood cells within the body. Melanocytes aid the protective mechanism against harmful rays of the sun by producing the brown melanin cells, which are stimulated on exposure to ultraviolet light.

The dermis or 'true skin' is a strong protective mesh of thick protein collagen fibres, which make the skin tougher, with thinner but strong supporting reticular fibres and elastic fibres to provide flexibility. The dermis also contains blood vessels which, in aromatherapy, carry the fat-soluble essential oil molecules around the body, lymphatic vessels, nerve fibres, glands and hair follicles. The dermis is indefinably divided into a papillary and a reticular layer. The papillary layer is composed of loose connective tissue with bundles of collagenous fibres. It has tiny, fine papillae joining it to the epidermal ridges, which are unique to the individual. Capillaries within the papillae nourish the epidermis and the special touch receptors known as Meissner's corpuscles. The reticular layer of dense connective tissue has a mesh of collagenous fibre bundles which form a strong elastic network with a dominant directional pattern in different areas of the body. Tension lines in the skin resulting from this directional pattern of the fibres are called Langer's or cleavage lines. Surgical incisions made parallel to the cleavage lines promote more rapid healing and less scarring than when an incision crosses the lines. Overstretching of the dermis during pregnancy can lead to tearing of the elastic and collagen fibres, with the repairing scar tissue resulting in striae gravidarum. Also within the reticular layer are blood and lymphatic vessels, nerves and free nerve endings, fat cells, sebaceous glands and hair roots. Deep muscle receptors called Pacinian corpuscles are also found in this layer and in the subcuticular hypodermal layer. Muscle fibres are present too in the reticular layer of the genital area and nipples. The subcutaneous hypodermis of loose fibrous connective adipose tissue is thick and has a rich supply of blood vessels, lymphatics and nerves, as well as the bases of the hair follicles and the sweat glands. Figure 3.1 shows the structure of the skin.

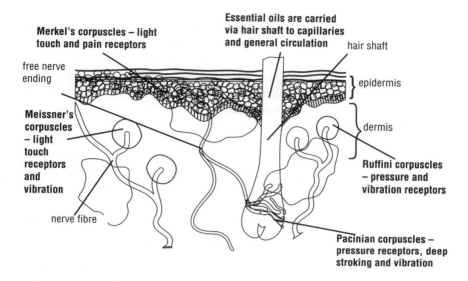

Figure 3.1 Structure of skin showing touch receptors

Absorption of essential oils through the epidermis and dermis is facilitated by transport down the hair shafts, and from there into the capillaries and the general circulation. Transport of essential oils also occurs between and through the skin cells. In some parts of the body there are thick layers of adipose cells – for example in the breasts and on the abdomen. The most permeable areas of the skin for the passage of essential oil molecules are the soles, palms, forehead, scalp and axillae. Hirsute areas of the body also facilitate the passage of essential oil molecules but the legs, abdomen and trunk are less permeable. The carrier oil used will also affect the rate of absorption, with many of the thicker, more viscous carriers (e.g. wheatgerm or avocado oil) impairing the rate, although those rich in polyunsaturates are absorbed fairly quickly. However, volatility of the essential oil molecules may be decreased by a particular carrier, thereby affecting absorption rates, or the skin enzymes may trigger molecular metabolism of certain constituents. The P450 skin enzymes, which aid detoxification of poisons, making them more soluble prior to urinary excretion, chemically alter some essential oils. In some cases, as with the contraindicated pennyroyal oil, this can result in the production of substances which can be extremely toxic.

A variety of sensations are perceived by the skin, due to the presence of sensory receptors. The sense of touch is actually a response to three stimuli – pressure, temperature and pain. Light touch, without indentation of the skin surface, is detected in the dermis by the free nerve endings and Meissner's corpuscles, and in the epidermis of the soles and palms by free nerve endings and Merkel's corpuscles. Deeper pressure results in temporary indentation of the skin and is detected by Pacinian corpuscles, the mechanoreceptors situated in the dermal and subcutaneous layers, which measure pressure changes. Variable vibrations of the skin, as with some of the percussion movements used in massage, are detected by Pacinian corpuscles, Meissner's corpuscles and the Ruffini corpuscles, depending on the frequency and depth of vibration. Naked nerve endings can measure heat and cold, while specialised free nerve endings throughout the body are sensitive to different types of pain. Continuous low-key stimulation of slow-conducting nerve fibres, mainly in the superficial layers of the skin, is thought to be the mechanism by which itches and ticklish sensations are perceived – these will be activated if massage pressure is significantly too light. The sensory neural pathways to the brain for both light touch and pain are situated in the spinothalamic tract ending in the cerebral cortex, which is why light effleurage or stroking can act as a means of easing pain.

Different types of massage stimulate different sensory receptors, which aim to help restore or maintain homeostasis. Light touch stimulates the Meissner's corpuscles and type 1 cutaneous mechanoreceptors, as well as the root hair nerve plexuses and free nerve endings. Deep stroking and compression techniques stimulate the pressure receptors, Pacinian corpuscles and type 2 cutaneous mechanoreceptors. Field, Diego and Hernandex-Reif (2010) found that moderate to deep pressure is required for massage to have any real physiological effects since this increases vagal activity, bringing about the recognised benefits of massage. This study supported the earlier findings of Morelli, Chapman and Sullivan (1999), who postulated that deep mechanoreceptors were involved in any physiological reactions to massage.

Manipulation of the skin during massage also stimulates the sebaceous glands and creates warmth, causing vasodilatation, increasing cell nutrition and an improvement in the general condition of the skin. Venous return and general circulation are enhanced, and blood pressure is temporarily reduced. The oxygen-carrying capacity of the blood is increased, lymphatic circulation improves and elimination processes are accelerated. It is thought that massage can aid the immune system by encouraging an increase in natural killer cells. Soft tissues, particularly the muscles, can be relaxed. Massage also has a marked effect on the nervous system, including relief of pain through the gate control mechanism (Melzack and Wall 1965), and an increase in alpha and delta wave activity in the brain, the former being associated with relaxation and the latter with inducing sleep. There is also a reduction in beta wave activity which is associated with mental alertness and stress. Vibrational movements such as tapotement (tapping) stimulate the Pacinian corpuscles, while manipulative movements stretch the tissues and muscle fibres. Stretching and other movements facilitated by the practitioner stimulate the proprioceptors in skeletal muscle, tendons and joints. Massage also stimulates the parasympathetic nervous system, promoting relaxation and reducing stress through a rise in dopamine and serotonin. Increased parasympathetic activity stimulates intestinal peristalsis, while the capillary circulation and lymphatic drainage increase urine output. Finally, the thermoreceptors detect hot and cold stimuli.

Measurement of pressure is now possible using various new technologies (Tee *et al.* 2015) or magnetic resonance imaging (Gay *et al.* 2014). Wu *et al.* (2014) demonstrated significant positive changes in electroencephalogram monitoring and in cortisol levels of subjects who received periodic aromatherapy massage, although it is difficult to elucidate whether the massage or the specific oils used were responsible for these effects.

Massage enhances the rate of systemic absorption of essential oils due to the increased blood flow. Certain oils, such as tea tree and peppermint, may affect the absorption of other, more harmful substances although this does seem to be dose-dependent (Nielsen 2006; Nielsen and Nielsen 2006). However, whilst it may be assumed that a warm room, warm client, warm oils and the warm hands of the practitioner could increase absorption of the oils, it is probable that the molecules are also readily vaporised and are therefore inhaled, with any physiological effects being due to a combination of absorption via the skin and via the respiratory tract (see Box 3.1).

Box 3.1 Physiological effects of massage

Stimulates circulation, aids oxygen-carrying capacity of blood vessels.

Stimulates sebaceous glands and aids vasodilatation.

Increases vagal activity.

Accelerates excretion.

Aids lymphatic drainage.

Reduces blood pressure.

Boosts immune system.

Eases pain via gate control mechanism.

Relaxes muscles:

- – Aids relaxation and induces sleep.
- – Reduces beta wave activity to reduce stress.

Administration of essential oils via inhalation

Inhalation of essential oil molecules occurs with every aromatherapy treatment, irrespective of the primary method of administration (see Chapter 2). Anyone exposed to the aroma will inhale some of the volatile essential oil molecules from the air via the nostrils, which then pass via the olfactory system to be perceived as an aroma, as well as via the respiratory tract to the general circulation. As has been discussed elsewhere (see Chapter 4) the client receiving aromatherapy is not the only person present who will inhale the chemicals from the essential oils –the practitioner and anyone else in contact with the mother will also be affected.

Olfaction is closely associated with taste, and much of what we taste is actually smell. Smells are detected first by inhaling an odour via the nostrils. The two nasal cavities are lined with mucus membrane and moistened by mucus secretions, into which chemicals entering the nose must dissolve before they can be detected. A small area in the upper nasal cavity contains the olfactory cells, and molecules from the aroma must bind to the sensory receptors in these cells. The olfactory mucus contains odour-binding proteins which dissolve the aroma molecules and increase its concentration in the mucus relative to inhaled air. The odour-binding proteins also remove 'used' aromas, which are then broken down, and free up the receptors to detect new aromatic molecules. Binding of the aroma alters the receptor structure and activates an olfactory protein which converts to adenosine triphosphate (ATP), which in turns converts to a substance called cyclic adenosine monophosphate (cAMP). The cAMP opens ion channels, depolarising the receptors through an electrical trigger of a nerve impulse. Impulses from the nasal receptors are then sent along the olfactory nerve (the first cranial nerve) to the brain.

Cranial nerves that transport impulses to the brain are sensory; those that carry impulses away from the brain are motor nerves. Sensory information from the nasal olfactory receptors is carried to the olfactory bulb in the front of the brain, into the area called the rhinencephalon. The olfactory tract connects to the neocortex, enabling recognition of aromas based on previous experiences. Also in this area of the brain is the limbic system, which is directly linked to the olfactory system. The limbic system is perhaps the most primitive part of the human brain and is thought to be the seat of the emotions and of memory. The septal nuclei and the amygdala are aroused when exposed to pleasant sensations, and the hippocampus is related to memory. It is interesting to note that even in people with no sense of smell (anosmia) the psychological effects of essential oils are still experienced (Chioca *et al.* 2013), although some people with anosmia can experience severe psycho-emotional upheaval due to a reduced impact on the amygdala.

Perception of aromas is an experience unique to each individual. Acceptance of an aroma oil blend is subjective and based on anticipation (Köteles and Babulka 2014), past exposure and experiences, and different aromas can often elicit long-forgotten memories through the stimulation of the amygdala and the hippocampus. There is even some suggestion, from animal research, that aromatic olfactory experiences in pregnancy can have an epigenetic effect, influencing behaviour in the offspring (Dias and Ressler 2014). Mental images may play a part in aroma perception, although anosmics appear better able to self-evaluate smell performance through the use of visual images (Kollndorfer *et al.* 2015). Aromas are known to have an impact on mood, through an effect on the prefrontal cortex of the brain. Igarashi *et al.* (2014) demonstrated significant changes in various parameters, including a decrease in oxyhaemoglobin and an increase in pleasurable feelings and uplifting of the mood, in subjects exposed to rose and orange oil.

Inhalation of essential oils via the nostrils also transfers the aromatic molecules to the respiratory tract via the nasopharynx, the trachea and thence to the lungs via the bronchi. Within the lungs, the bronchi divide into a 'respiratory tree' and finally into the bronchioles, ending in the microscopic alveoli, the air sacs in which gaseous exchange occurs. Each lung contains over 350 million alveoli surrounded by capillaries which have extremely thin walls, allowing for the diffusion of oxygen and carbon dioxide between them. Once in the blood vessels, oxygen and any other molecules carried with it are transported around the body, partially in solution and partially with haemoglobin, to be used as required.

It is obvious that for some conditions involving the cardiorespiratory system, such as colds and sinus congestion, administration of essential oils by inhalation could be the treatment method of choice, while congestion of the mucus membranes will slow down systemic absorption. Certain essential oils will have an immediate effect on the respiratory tract, particularly those which are high in ketones (see page 72) and the oxide 1.8 cineole. Other oils, such as eucalyptus and frankincense, are known to have significant decongestant and mucolytic effects due to activation of the cilia in the nostrils as the aroma (chemicals) is inhaled. However, the fact that essential oils can be transported systemically makes inhalation a valuable method for treatment of other conditions, particularly as it is thought that certain essential oils have an affinity for particular organs. For example, original research by Falk-Filipsson *et al.* (1993) suggested that monoterpenes are very soluble in blood and have a high respiratory uptake, and demonstrated approximately 70% pulmonary uptake of limonene after inhalation. Figures 3.2a and 3.2b show the anatomical structures involved when essential oils are inhaled.

a.

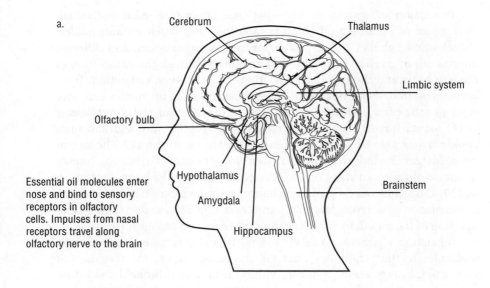

Cerebrum

Thalamus

Limbic system

Olfactory bulb

Hypothalamus

Brainstem

Amygdala

Hippocampus

Essential oil molecules enter nose and bind to sensory receptors in olfactory cells. Impulses from nasal receptors travel along olfactory nerve to the brain

b.

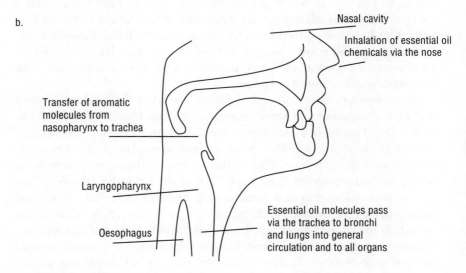

Nasal cavity

Inhalation of essential oil chemicals via the nose

Transfer of aromatic molecules from nasopharynx to trachea

Laryngopharynx

Oesophagus

Essential oil molecules pass via the trachea to bronchi and lungs into general circulation and to all organs

Figure 3.2 Anatomical structures involved when essential oils are inhaled

Chemistry of essential oils

Essential oils contain numerous chemical constituents, each of which has a particular odour and will have a particular physiological and/or psychological effect on specific cells, dependent on their structure. Most essential oils contain similar constituents, or derivatives of a primary group of constituents, but the proportions of each constituent will be different in each different oil. A typical essential oil will contain around 200 different constituents, although when looking at the chemical profile of an essential oil, those constituents listed first will be in the highest proportions, whereas those in minute amounts are usually not listed at all. Trace constituents will be present in minute amounts in some oils – for example, 1.8 cineole is found in both eucalyptus and mandarin oils, but while it is a major component of the former, it may be up to 40,000 times less in the latter (Tisserand and Young 2014).

Factors such as climate, altitude, seasons and other growing conditions for the plant will affect the proportion of individual chemical constituents in the essential oils, within a given range. For example, high-altitude lavender from Austria or Switzerland is much purer than lavender grown at lower altitudes and has a more distinctive aroma (and is thus more expensive). Some constituents will occur in higher proportions in the essential oil at certain times of the year, such as the menthone content of mint oils, which may be higher in the summer and lower in the autumn. The process of extraction can also influence the constituents – for example, chamazulene, the constituent of chamomile essential oil which gives it its rich blue colour, is not found in the plant itself but is produced during the extraction process. Plants which have been subjected to spraying with pesticides may also contain traces of these sprays, particularly cold-pressed citrus oils. However, most of these substances are poorly absorbed through the skin so will not generally be a problem when essential oils are administered via massage, and the issue is more pertinent to oral administration, which is not permissible in maternity aromatherapy (see Chapters 2 and 4).

Unintentional contamination with phthalates or intentional adulteration may occasionally be found in certain essential oils. Adulteration involves the deliberate addition of substances to increase the yield (and therefore profits) by diluting the original concentrated essential oil, most commonly those which are expensive, such as jasmine, rose, ylang ylang and neroli. These added substances may be other similar-smelling essential oils – for example, rose geranium is occasionally added to the much more expensive rose oil, or the adulterant may consist of other aromatic or non-aromatic compounds. Where a substance has been added, this should be listed on the label. Rose or jasmine oil, for example, may legitimately have a small amount of fractionated coconut oil added (usually 5%) to stabilise it and to enable practitioners to harness the benefits of the oil without the expense of one which is usually produced as an absolute, used mainly in the perfumery industry and rarely used in clinical aromatherapy. Conversely, unscrupulous producers may add synthetic substances to an essential oil without declaring it – this is why it is so important to purchase good-quality essential oils from a reputable supplier.

Deterioration of essential oils occurs over time, although this process can be expedited by poor storage or exposure of the oil to the air (oxidisation). Essential oils which are rich in monoterpenes tend to deteriorate more rapidly than some others, while unsaturated oils become rancid and exude a noticeably different aroma than when the oil is fresh. Oxidised essential oils undergo a change in their chemical composition which may affect the efficacy and even become hazardous. For example, essential oils may lose their antibacterial effect as they deteriorate, and those containing high levels of terpenes may cause an increased risk of skin irritation. Oils which are rich in limonene are particularly susceptible to this. Inappropriate storage will exacerbate this process, so citrus oils, which contain large proportions of limonene, should be stored at temperatures below 5°C. Tea tree oil rich in 1.8 cineole will deteriorate less rapidly than tea tree with lower concentrations. Excessive heat can also cause deterioration in some essential oils, so even those which do not need to be kept in a refrigerator should be stored at ambient temperatures. Prolonged exposure to ultraviolet light will potentially cause an increase in some chemical constituents and a decrease in others, significantly altering the overall chemical composition and making the oils unsuitable for clinical use. Other substances which come into contact with pure essential oils, such as resins or plastics, will expedite oxidisation. The addition of water (two parts hydrogen and one part oxygen) promotes oxidisation, molecular hydrolysis and discolouration of the essential oils. Interestingly, although it is generally held in clinical practice that blended essential oils lead to early deterioration, it has been suggested that combining certain essential oils, without carrier oil, can actually prolong 'shelf life', although this is not to be recommended in maternity aromatherapy until more is known about this aspect (Misharina and Polshkov 2005). (See also Chapter 2 for the clinical application related to oxidisation.)

All essential oils are organic matter formed as a result of the combination of the chemical element carbon with hydrogen and oxygen atoms, and occasionally also with nitrogen and sulphur. Combined carbon and hydrogen atoms (hydrocarbons) and oxygenated hydrocarbons (with the addition of oxygen) form the main components of essential oils, with other functional groups attached, including alcohols, esters, aldehydes, ketones and phenols. Other substances, such as tannins, mucilages and flavonoids, plant constituents used therapeutically in herbal medicine, are not found in essential oils, because extraction of the oils usually involves water, so that only small, volatile, water-insoluble substances can be isolated from the plant. Hydrocarbons are, however, soluble in lipids, which is one of the reasons why a carrier oil is usually used when blending essential oils for clinical practice.

Hydrocarbons vary in molecular size and complexity, the more complex being more easily oxidised when the chemical bonds are broken. The most commonly occurring hydrocarbons are terpenoids, which give rise to the chemical group called terpenes. Terpenes are formed of isoprene units, which build up to make the sub-groups of terpenes found in essential oils. Monoterpenes are formed of two isoprene units, sesquiterpenes have three isoprene units and diterpenes consist of four isoprene units. Chemical constituents which are part of the terpene group have names ending in 'ene', such as limonene, occurring in citrus oils including bergamot, sweet orange, lime and lemon oils, as well as peppermint, although terpenes are found to a greater or lesser extent in all essential oils. Monoterpenes have strongly antibacterial and analgesic properties and may also be decongestant and expectorant and have a stimulating effect (Guimarães, Quintans and Quintans 2013). Sesquiterpenes are antibacterial, anti-inflammatory, relaxing and hypotensive, with some also being analgesic and antispasmodic. Diterpenes occur less frequently in essential oils as they have a higher molecular weight than mono- and sesquiterpenes and a higher boiling point, which prevents them from being extracted from the plant when steam distillation is used (see Chapter 2 for methods of extraction). Those diterpenes which do occur in essential oils are said to be antifungal and antiviral, expectorant and possibly to have a balancing effect on the hormones. Most essential oil constituents are derived from terpenes or terpinoid molecules, but the method of extraction affects the proportion of terpenes in the extracted oils. Cold expression, a squeezing process used to extract citrus essences, facilitates transfer of terpenes so that citrus oils may have up to 90% of substances such as limonene. Conversely, solvent extraction and some of the newer methods of obtaining essential oils or absolutes from delicate plants such as rose contain minimal amounts of terpenes.

Alcohol functional groups include monoterpenols (in which the alcohol is attached to a terpene) such as geraniol (found in geranium) and linalool (found in lavender) – the names ending in 'ol'. However, caution must be employed when reviewing chemical names, since those in another group, phenols, also have names ending in 'ol'. Alcohols are the most varied type of terpene derivatives and are considered to be the most therapeutically beneficial component of essential oils, with low toxicity and pleasant flowery aromas. These substances are also antibacterial and antiviral, they are uplifting and warming and are generally thought, in clinical aromatherapy, to be balancing to both physical and emotional health.

Phenols are superficially chemically similar to alcohols but should be viewed with caution in clinical practice since they are well known to cause skin irritation. Phenols are one of the main ingredients found in cleaning solutions and have a strong antiseptic action but may also be stimulating to the immune and nervous systems. A phenol compound, eugenol, is found in ylang ylang and rose essential oils, but these two oils are not generally considered to cause skin irritation when used in suitably diluted doses – presumably because the proportion of eugenol to other constituents is minimal. A slight chemical variation on phenols is the group of phenolic ethers, including constituents such as anethole, safrole and methyl chavicol (estragole), all of which are potentially toxic, with some evidence of carcinogenicity and abortifacient properties. (See Chapter 4 for the safety of essential oils.)

Aldehydes occur widely in essential oils and are possibly partially oxidised primary alcohols. They are formed when carbon atoms are joined by a hydrogen atom and a carboxyl group (carbon and oxygen linked by a double bond) but are not within a carbonic chain. The double bond means that aldehydes break down relatively easily so they will oxidise quickly. As oxidisation occurs, aldehydes are converted into acids which can be astringent and often act as a catalyst for other chemical reactions. Their names end in 'al' – for example, geranial (found in geranium) – or 'aldehyde'. A commonly known aldehyde is formaldehyde, although this compound is not found in essential oils. Aldehydes tend to smell quite sharp – for example, the aroma of almonds in sweet almond carrier oil is due to the presence of benzyl aldehyde, responsible for the rapid oxidisation which can occur (and to which 1% of the population is allergic). Aldehydes are calming and sedative, and can reduce blood pressure and temperature through a vasodilator effect. Although they have some anti-infective capability, it is not as strong as in alcohols and ketones. Some aldehydes are also skin irritants, notably citral found in bergamot oil.

Ketones are structurally similar to aldehydes and are sometimes produced by oxidisation of secondary alcohols, although they are fairly stable compounds and do not readily oxidise further. They are not easily metabolised in the human body and may be excreted via the kidneys unchanged. Generally, the names end in 'one', such as carvone (found in spearmint oil) or menthone (found in mint oils), although the proportion of ketones in these oils is much lower than other chemical constituents. One exception to the 'one' rule is camphor, a ketone found in rosemary, sage and certain lavender-type oils (but not common lavender, *Lavandula angustifolia*). Ketones are calming and sedative, analgesic, mucolytic and expectorant, and appear to have an effect on the digestive system. On the other hand, some essential oils contain high levels of ketones, such as pinocamphone, in hyssop oil, and pulegone, in pennyroyal oil, both of which can be neurotoxic, leading to epileptiform convulsions and other problems (see Chapter 4). Other essential oils relatively high in ketones include jasmine and sweet fennel, suitable for use during or after labour, and thuja and wormwood which are contraindicated in clinical aromatherapy.

Esters are formed when an acid and an alcohol combine; they form the most widespread group of compounds in essential oils and fragrances. The names of esters end in 'ate' or 'acetate'. They are considered generally safe with low toxicity, except methyl salicylate and sabinyl acetate found in Spanish sage oil. Examples of esters include benzyl acetate, a floral, fruity aroma occurring in jasmine, neroli and ylang ylang, and linalyl acetate in bergamot, lavender, clary sage and neroli oils. Esters are strongly sedative, anti-inflammatory and antispasmodic. Certain types of chamomile essential oil can have up to 60% esters in their chemical make-up, resulting in chamomile being very effective in aiding sleep, promoting wound healing and reducing gastrointestinal spasm.

Other constituents found in essential oils in lower proportions than those outlined above include lactones, furanocoumarins and oxides. Lactones are only found in small amounts in expressed oils and some absolutes (e.g. jasmine) and may have expectorant and antipyretic properties. Furanocoumarins occur in citrus oils, particularly bergamot, which must always be diluted, and to a lesser extent in lemon, sweet orange and mandarin/tangerine. They have a reputation for being phototoxic (see Chapter 4), possibly through the interference with melanin-producing skin cells. They may also have an anticoagulant effect, although this tends to be related more to phytocoumarins used in herbal medicine, and to be hypotensive and uplifting. Oxides occur in essential oils and have a camphorous aroma (e.g. eucalyptus, tea tree and rosemary). The most commonly found oxide in essential oils used in clinical aromatherapy is eucalyptol, also known as 1.8 cineole, which is strongly expectorant.

Pharmacokinetics of essential oils

Bioavailability refers to the proportion of an administered dose of a substance which reaches the systemic circulation, and depends on the substance, the method, dose and frequency of administration. Bioavailability will be affected by the individual recipient, including their general health and wellbeing, age, ethnicity, metabolism and factors such as the environment, hirsutism and skin integrity. In general aromatherapy practice, gender is also a factor.

When essential oils are administered via the skin, absorption rates differ between individuals, between different areas of the body and between chemical constituents. Whilst the skin allows for slower absorption than the gastrointestinal tract, the fact that the skin is the body's largest organ means that there will, overall, be considerable absorption and systemic circulation. The carrier medium used for massage – usually a vegetable oil – results in slower absorption than when essential oils are added to water, particularly when the water is hot, which causes vasodilatation and opens up the hair shafts. However, massage stimulates the local circulation, which aids absorption, although essential oils which are more volatile will evaporate into the air quickly, reducing the amount available for dermal absorption. Applying essential oils to warm skin, either in water or as a massage, will also enhance absorption. Neat oil absorbs more quickly than essential oil diluted in carrier oil, due to percutaneous absorption, and results in higher concentrations of the chemical constituents in the bloodstream, increasing the risk of toxicity (see Chapter 4). The essential oils mix with skin lipids, reducing the barrier function of the skin by making them more hydrophilic, and are therefore facilitated to cross into the dermal layer. Trauma to the skin and dermatitis conditions such as eczema or psoriasis reduce the skin integrity and allow faster absorption of essential oils, and the resulting immune response may cause inflammation. Even stress can affect the ability of the skin to absorb essential oils appropriately, either expediting or inhibiting absorption. Although most essential oil constituents will be fully absorbed into the circulation within 24 hours, some will be retained for up to 72 hours in the epidermis before crossing to the dermis and then into the systemic circulation. There is some suggestion that human skin is more permeable in the evenings and at night rather than in the morning (Yosipovitch et al. 1998), and pigmented skin appears to have a better barrier function, implying slower absorption than in pale-skinned women. Covering the skin after administration may also encourage greater absorption.

Neonatal skin is much thinner than adult skin and dermal application should be completely avoided until at least three months of age. It is not the purpose of this book to consider aromatherapy in babies, but midwives and doulas should be mindful of these issues and take steps to advise women accordingly. Tisserand and Young (2014) suggest that children aged 3–24 months should receive no more than 0.25%; for those aged 2–6 years a maximum of 1% is recommended; 1.5% is advised for children up to the age of 15 years. Any commercial products intended for infants should only contain essential oils if they have been dispersed in a water-soluble medium.

Essential oils administered via inhalation pass to the respiratory tract and reach the pulmonary alveoli, which facilitate the passage of the small molecules into the bloodstream and subsequently pass into the central nervous system (CNS) relatively quickly. This has implications for women with CNS conditions such as epilepsy (see Chapter 4). There is only a single membrane for the lipophilic molecules to traverse into the lungs, so inhalation of essential oils can produce a substantial – and possibly an adverse – reaction. Even inhaling vapours from adding essential oils to the bath water can have a crucial effect. Entry via the blood–brain barrier can also be significant. The rate and depth of breathing influences absorption, so women in the transition stage of labour, who may be hyperventilating, will absorb more essential oil than when they are breathing normally. Prolonged exposure to vapours (more than 30 minutes) may not only trigger the minor side-effects associated with the aromas but may also have more widespread systemic effects. When essential oils are administered via inhalation, whether as the primary method or as a secondary effect of dermal administration, it is difficult to assess the dosage. This is particularly so when certain constituents are more volatile than others and are more rapidly lost to the atmosphere.

Essential oils are lipophilic and, once absorbed into the body, generally work in a similar way to other fat-soluble substances. Distribution of essential oils in the general circulation depends on the degree of their lipophilic activity. Essential oil constituents penetrate the blood–brain barrier and can have a direct effect on various receptors in the brain. They also reach the liver and kidneys rapidly, whereas their impact on skeletal muscle is less significant. Essential oils will be stored in adipose tissue for some considerable time, depending on the oil and its various constituents, during which time they have little or no pharmacological action. Retention of the oil chemicals in the fat will obviously be considerable in obese women and significantly less so in those who have a very low body mass index.

Essential oil molecules which have metabolised will eventually bind to plasma-binding proteins in the same way as drugs. This inactivates any further pharmacological action, but the molecules can also not be transformed and excreted, essentially prolonging their retention by the body. Interaction with drugs competing for the same protein-binding sites may also occur. However, this is not a major issue when essential oils are administered in clinically appropriate doses via the skin or inhalation, and refers more significantly to oral or even intravenous administration. However, some essential oil constituents raise the production of metabolic enzymes which may increase or decrease the rate of metabolism and exacerbate the potential for drug–oil interaction. This is particularly the case with the cytochrome P450 enzyme found in the liver and small intestine, although essential oils would have to be administered in large doses, primarily via inhalation or by mouth, to have any real adverse effects (this is unlikely to occur with dermal administration). There is also a theoretical possibility of some essential oil constituents inhibiting or exacerbating other chemicals when present in large amounts. These include monoamine oxidase inhibitors, selective serotonin reuptake inhibitors, anticoagulants (e.g. warfarin and heparin) and tyramine, but the limited amount of evidence refers largely to oral administration and is not explored here. Despite this, there are anecdotal reports of pathological complications occurring when essential oils have been administered in people taking various drugs and it is wise to be extremely cautious when using aromatherapy for pregnant women with medical conditions for which they require medication (see Chapter 4).

Different rates of metabolism are seen with different chemical constituents which are eventually excreted via the kidneys, liver, lungs, skin and intestines. All essential oil constituents in the bloodstream pass through the kidneys and are excreted in the urine but, for those which adhere strongly to the plasma proteins, filtration and excretion will be slower. Essential oils which are inhaled will be excreted only in very small amounts by the kidneys, pulmonary excretion being the main method. Small amounts of some constituents may pass to the sweat, faeces, saliva and breastmilk, and in this latter case, can be ingested by the baby.

The concept of energy in aromatherapy

Aromatherapists and massage therapists often refer to the notion of energy transfer between the client and the practitioner. Although this can at first appear to be a rather nebulous concept, which has not, hitherto, sat comfortably within conventional medicine, there is a growing understanding of the principle of energetic transfer.

Kinetic energy within the body is, essentially, heat. If one considers the simple activity of sitting on a cold chair, we can appreciate that, after some time, the chair will warm up as a result of body heat being transferred to the seat. In other words, the positive (warm) energy of the person has been transferred by a process of conduction to overcome the negative (cold) energy of the chair seat.

During pregnancy, the increased cell mass from the developing fetus and extra circulating fluid raises the overall metabolism of the mother and baby unit, producing more energy as a by-product, naturally increasing the body temperature by around 1°C. This heat circulates via the blood to the skin from where it is lost through normal homeostatic processes. Stress, pain and illness accelerate internal body functioning, thus producing even more heat.

During massage, there is an increase in heat, both in the skin of the client and the hands of the therapist, with the amount of kinetic energy depending on pressure (weight) and speed. The type of massage techniques employed also affect heat, with faster, deeper movements producing more energy, thereby increasing skin and core temperature further. Scientists at McMaster University in Canada used gene-profiling techniques to demonstrate molecular changes resulting from the heat generated by post-exercise massage, including a reduction in inflammatory cytokines and an increase in recovery of over-worked muscle groups. The study found that massage appears to activate some genes which reduce inflammation, acting as a natural pain reliever, and others which generate mitochondria, helping the cells to take up and use oxygen. The authors of the study suggest that the heat produced during massage suppresses the inflammatory response and facilitates the recovery process (Crane *et al.* 2012). Conversely, traditional ice-bath techniques for reducing muscle soreness, originally thought to reduce the inflammatory response, may in fact block muscle repair and growth, possibly due to the reduced electrical impulse conduction which occurs in water.

The human body is actually surrounded by an energy field which extends beyond the physical boundaries of the skin. This can be experienced as warmth emanating from rubbing one's hands together vigorously. When the two hands are separated then slowly brought together again, warmth and a slight pressure between the hands can be felt, indicating the energy field as both hands meet in the middle. The depth of the energy field varies according to homeostatic balance, either increasing or decreasing from the norm in times of physical or emotional stress or dis-ease.

The earth also has an electrical energy field, as does the sun. Incoming radiation from the sun hits the earth and is absorbed by the ionospheric layer, which resonates at an energy level of 7.83 Hz. Humans (and animals and objects) on the earth act as a conduit between the earth and the sun. It has been suggested that when the energy of an individual is the same as that of the sun and the earth (7.83 Hz), the person is in optimal health, but stressors (illness) alter the energy, causing an imbalance. This concept of the interaction of the energies was identified by the German professor Winfried Otto Schumann in 1952 and is known as Schumann resonance (Schumann and Konig 1952). Some people believe that Schumann resonance protects us from the harmful rays of the sun, but electro-magnetic (kinetic) energy, such as that from radio waves, will adversely affect the person's energy level. Naturally occurring energy changes, including volcanoes, natural gas emissions or electrical storms, can also affect Schumann resonance, leading to changes in health and wellbeing. This is called geopathic stress.

There is increasing concern about the impact of man-made geopathic stress from technology, including wireless internet, mobile telephones, microwave ovens, etc., on human health. The heat produced from electrical equipment can be transferred into the body, especially when in direct contact, such as with a mobile phone. The electrical energy waves are transferred via the ear, impacting on brain waves and thus altering the body's energy balance. If the phone is kept in a trouser pocket, the energy is transferred to the pelvic region, potentially affecting the gonads and reducing fertility, especially in men. Chronic energy imbalance adversely affects numerous physical and mental processes, leading to a lowered immune system, depression, dementia, etc. and has been shown adversely to affect heart rate and blood pressure (Dharmadhikari *et al.* 2010; Saunders 2003).

Many complementary therapies harness the concept of energy. Reiki practitioners use techniques designed to re-balance homeostasis by 'massaging' the energetic field (sometimes called the 'aura') around the body.

Kinesiology is a diagnostic technique in which assessment of muscle energy (heat) helps to detect issues such as food intolerances, or allergies to non-organic substances. Homeopathic remedies are claimed to be energised through a process of dilution and succession (shaken vigorously) which releases energy from the remedy material into the water. The more the original substance is diluted and succussed (shaken vigorously), the more energetic (i.e. powerful) the final homeopathic remedy becomes physically, rather than chemically. Indeed, the fragile chemical nature of homeopathic remedies means that they should not be stored near essential oils with their greater chemical energy, nor near equipment which emits electrical energy waves such as mobile telephones.

Traditional Chinese medicine (TCM) uses the concept of opposing principles, including Yin and Yang, which refer to energy transfer along superficial channels connecting one part of the body to another. Yin is cool or reduced energy whilst Yang is hot or active energy, with individual homeostasis depending on having a reasonable balance between the two. The principles of the Yin–Yang balance can be applied to conventional physiology – for example, testosterone is active (Yang) whereas oestrogen is gentler (Yin). In relation to massage, percussion and fast, deep petrissage movements are Yang, but gentle, slow, light effleurage is Yin, as is holding and pausing during the treatment. In TCM terms, this is one reason why it is important to use a variety of massage techniques within the treatment in order to restore the client's Yin–Yang balance.

Energy transfer between the practitioner and the client is important in manual therapy. The therapist absorbs energy from the client and needs to dissipate this heat. If the mother's condition is compromised by pain or stress, her energy will not be functioning at the optimum 7.83 Hz. It is to be hoped that the midwife or other practitioner will be in good health with an energy level of around 7.83 Hz, allowing for positive energy to be transferred to the mother to help her regain a homeostatically normal energy level. Trying to provide a treatment when the midwife is tired, over-worked, irritable or developing a cold alters her own energy field and this somewhat more negative energy will then be transferred to the mother. Consequently, the midwife may actually feel better at the end of performing a massage because she has absorbed some of the mother's slightly more positive energy.

It is possible to limit the impact of any negative energy by 'grounding' oneself before commencing treatment. This involves working with the feet, preferably without shoes, in contact with the floor, to co-ordinate with the Schumann resonance between the earth and the sun. Some therapists like to focus on eliminating any negative emotions they may be feeling at the time, by imagining a barrier such as being inside a bubble, which protects the therapist from outside negative energies. If the mother is emitting negative energy, the practitioner can imagine her in another bubble, which is separate from their own. An example would be the mother who is so anxious that she becomes slightly aggressive, essentially preventing absorption of positive healing energy from the therapist. Sometimes a midwife will experience symptoms similar to those felt by the mother during the treatment – for example, a sensation of nausea or a twinge of pain. Another consequence of performing manual therapy without adequate protection of one's energy field could be extreme exhaustion out of proportion to the duration of the treatment. At the end of a treatment it is good practice for the therapist to wash their hands, not only from a hygiene perspective but in order to 'shake off' the energies which have been transmitted from the client. This is vital if another client is due to attend for treatment, in order to avoid the transfer of energy from one client to another.

Healing reactions which the mother may experience during or after therapy, such as crying or increased sweating (warm body fluids) or diuresis (raised energy levels), are the body's way of ridding itself of excess heat to re-energise the body towards homeostatic balance. Conversely, shaking and shivering during treatment is the natural response of the body to being cold.

Some aromatherapists focus strongly on the energy concept to enhance their practice, perhaps dowsing to determine the most appropriate essential oils to use for a particular client, or incorporating reiki into the treatment. Even when practice is not consciously focused on using energy, there is a natural energy transfer occurring. Patricia Davies, a well-known aromatherapy authority in the 1980s, wrote of 'subtle aromatherapy' in which she advocated using some of the more esoteric concepts to aid practice, including chakra balancing, dowsing, meditation and other Eastern practices (Davies 1991). The lack of an evidence base on these aspects of complementary medicine reinforced the belief at that time that aromatherapy and other therapies were akin to witchcraft. More recently, advances in scientific research, both directly related to complementary medicine and in the field of quantum physics, have started to dispel these myths and to give modalities such as aromatherapy, massage and reflexology a more robust theoretical underpinning.

Touch and healing are an inherent part of the human experience and the body's natural energy field can be influenced positively through massage. We touch people to nurture them, to console them in times of need and to reduce pain by rubbing an injured part of the body. Touch is a form of communication and to be touched is a basic human need. Research has shown that elderly people who are not regularly touched by someone can deteriorate emotionally and physically. Studies on preterm infants have shown increased growth, weight gain, development and maturity when they have received regular massage, possibly through an impact on vagal activity (Diego, Field and Hernadez-Reif 2014). Touch has been shown to increase alpha brain waves, producing a state of relaxation similar to meditation, together with a lowering of cortisol (Rudnicki et al. 2012; Wu et al. 2014).

Essential oils also possess an energetic capacity, the precise frequencies (Hz measurement) varying between oils. Some of the early work on the energetic principles of essential oils was undertaken by the French essential oil chemist, Michel Lavabre (1990), although Peace Rhind (2012) attributes the oil properties to functional molecular characteristics. This energy concept in relation to essential oils was originally propounded by Lavabre's 'evolution–involution' theory, in which he assumed that each plant evolves from the physical sphere (its grounding with the earth), its vital sphere with the leaves and its astral sphere with the flowers. Involution involves the production of fruit and seeds, a process which returns the plant to the soil to recommence the life cycle. For example, the cypress tree has a very long life, giving it an enduring and stabilising effect on the ground, and cypress essential oil is said to have similar properties in terms of balancing physical and mental equilibrium in clients. In energetic aromatherapy, black pepper essential oil is thermally warming, but is also warming to the spirit, helping to dispel negative emotions and thoughts. Peppermint, known to have a physiologically cooling effect on the skin, can also be used to calm and cool the mood in cases of agitation.

This area of aromatherapy has, as yet, no research evidence to support it, but is an interesting concept which some practitioners may wish to use alongside the chemical and physio-psychological approach. There is increasing investigation into the principle of energy in general, which may eventually lead us to studies on essential oil energetic characteristics in a more formal manner. In the meantime, an understanding of the concept of energy in relation to massage can be beneficial to therapy outcomes.

The difficulties of producing an evidence base for aromatherapy

Evidence-based practice is vital to the provision of safe, effective clinical care. Although some areas of conventional healthcare remain unevaluated, the culture of defensive practice to avoid litigation is so strong within obstetrics that it is essential to be able to argue the case for the efficacy and safety of aromatherapy in midwifery practice. Aromatherapists, too, who may have contact with midwives or obstetricians, need to be able to support their practice with research findings, in order to justify their actions.

Initially, the majority of essential oil research was undertaken mainly by the cosmetics and food industries, which explored the flavours and aromas, as well as the preservative qualities of the oils. More recently, considerable laboratory research has been conducted on the chemistry and clinical properties of individual oils – for example, the antibacterial effects of oils such as tea tree, one of the most commonly researched essential oils (Mertas *et al.* 2015; Warnke *et al.* 2013). Other research focuses on how aromatherapy works: is it due to the chemical constituents, the method of administration, particularly massage, or the therapeutic relationship between client and therapist?

Investigating single essential oils is acceptable to the medical and pharmaceutical professions, which view chemicals in isolation rather than as a part of the whole therapeutic event. Pharmaceutical companies spend many years and an enormous amount of money on clinical research and the development of new drugs. Since the thalidomide disaster of the 1960s, they are required to demonstrate beyond reasonable doubt that their products are safe for the public, and there are occasions when the potential side-effects on humans are found to be so unacceptable as to warrant discontinuation of the drug's development. The costs of this system, if applied to aromatherapy and herbal medicine, would be prohibitive, a fact which has been partly resolved through the 2011 EU laws on herbal medicines, which require registration of traditional remedies that have been in use for more than 30 years. Also, since it is not possible to patent natural products, there is no incentive for individual companies to undertake the research with all its accompanying costs, unless they can isolate the single active ingredient, synthesise it and then reproduce it and apply for a product patent. To a certain extent, this has some value in that essential oils and other herbal substances may be the precursors to some new drugs (Abd Kadir, Yaakob and Zulkifli 2013; Boukhatem *et al.* 2013), but adhering to the pharmaceutical approach does little to demonstrate the effectiveness and safety of aromatherapy as a clinical modality in its own right.

One of the problems for aromatherapy, as for other complementary therapies, is to demonstrate not only whether the essential oils are effective, but also how they work and whether they are safe, especially in pregnancy. The biomedical sciences have long seen randomised, double-blinded, controlled trials as the 'gold standard' by which all clinical studies should be measured. However, many complementary therapies cannot be investigated in this way because their effectiveness is based on factors that cannot be double-blinded, or treatment selections which must be individualised to each patient. In respect of aromatherapy, subjects could be randomly allocated to receive either an aromatherapy oil/treatment or a placebo/normal care, but studies cannot be double-blinded unless synthetically produced aromas are used in the control group, which in themselves may have some effect. Where massage is used as the method of administration, both the professional and the subject will, of course, be aware of the treatment, in which case a third subject group who receive essential oils via some other route, such as inhalation, will be necessary. There again, we have seen from the discussion in this chapter that there are physiological differences in the absorption of essential oils between dermal or respiratory administration, adding another complexity to the mix.

Many clinical applications of aromatherapy depend on a composite blend of different essential oils, usually administered via the skin in a massage or some other form of administration. In clinical practice, the aromatherapy treatment should be individualised for each client, and one blend of essential oils would not necessarily be appropriate for other individuals with the same symptoms or condition. There is now a trend in contemporary complementary medical research to study the effectiveness of the 'package' of care (i.e. treatment with aromatherapy) rather than its individual components – but this is contrary to the notion of randomised controlled trials, in which single specific aspects are investigated in order to eliminate confounding variables.

Whilst these problems also relate to many other complementary therapies, there are some issues which are pertinent to aromatherapy specifically. The chemistry of individual essential oils is influenced by factors such as geography, climate, the seasons, etc., so it is difficult to draw comparisons between studies which apparently use the same essential oils. For example, a study using 'lavender' could involve the use of high-altitude Alpine lavender or English lavender, which would have different proportions of the same chemical constituents, thus potentially affecting the results. In addition, there are several different types of some oils, so studies which apparently investigate 'chamomile' may, in fact, be using different oils with different chemical compositions – in this case, *Matricaria chamomilla* (German) or *Chamaemelum nobile* (Roman). Furthermore, the concept of psycho-aromatherapy adds another dimension to the picture: it is virtually impossible to eliminate the effects of aromas on the limbic centre of the brain when conducting trials of clinical aromatherapy.

Researching aromatherapy in a clinical setting is therefore complicated. There has, until recently, been little research on the use of aromatherapy in pregnancy and childbirth. What little clinical evidence there is tends to be based on the premise that the essential oils used are generally considered safe enough to use in pregnancy because there is no documented evidence to the contrary. Trials on the potential teratogenic or abortifacient effects of essential oils have been carried out only on animals such as mice, since it would be impossible to obtain ethical clearance to study these effects on pregnant women. However, it is difficult to relate animal physiology to human physiology, so the results can only act as a guide, particularly when the doses used in animal research are often many multiples of what would be considered suitable for clinical aromatherapy practice. Also, whilst humans generally have only one baby at a time, it is normal in animals to produce several offspring – a fact which may cause essential oils to have variable effects within and between litters. In some species, notably rodents, spontaneous fetal malformations are not uncommon, making it difficult to apportion blame when essential oils are administered. In addition, research animals are kept in a laboratory environment which is unnatural and it is not possible to determine whether the associated stress could have an additional impact on the development of embryonic and fetal malformations.

However, since it is impossible to conduct stringent testing for the safety of essential oils in human pregnancy, it is necessary to place some degree of reliance on animal testing. This means that, where a study has shown adverse effects in pregnant animals exposed to specific essential oils, it would be professionally expedient to avoid using this oil in pregnant humans. For example, Lis-Balchin, a chemist with an interest in essential oils, conducted research on rodents to examine safety in pregnancy. One of the essential oils, tea tree, was found potentially to relax smooth muscle, causing the researcher to comment in her final report that it would be unwise to use tea tree during (human) labour as it could theoretically have an adverse effect on the myometrium (Lis-Balchin 1999). In the absence of any more recent contradictory evidence, this then provides a guide to one essential oil, a fact that could be used by expert witnesses in the event of a case for alleged negligence during a labour in which tea tree had been used being brought to court for compensation.

The method of administration can also become a significant variable in aromatherapy studies. Massage in itself can be an effective therapeutic intervention. When combined with essential oils, the desired outcome may be enhanced, particularly in terms of relaxation, aiding sleep or easing pain. In order to conduct an aromatherapy study using robust research methodology, it would probably be necessary to have subjects randomly allocated to several groups: a control group, an essential oil group using inhalation as the method of administration, a massage group and a group in which both massage and the essential oils are used. For example, several studies have found inhalation of lavender to be effective as a sedative in those with sleep disturbances (Karadag et al. 2015; Keshavarz Afshar et al. 2015; Lillehei and Halcon 2014), whereas Hajibagheri, Babaii and Adib-Hajbaghery (2014) used rose oil in a massage treatment to aid sleep. Not only were different oils and administration methods used in these studies, but the clinical conditions also varied. Interestingly, Hwang and Shin's (2015) meta-analysis of several studies found that those involving inhalation of an essential oil were statistically more effective in inducing sleep than those which involved an aromatherapy massage treatment. It is therefore very difficult to determine with any degree of certainty whether or not 'aromatherapy' – or a specific essential oil – is useful in helping people get to sleep.

Obtaining evidence of the safety of aromatherapy is even more difficult, especially in pregnancy. Most of the information available about safety (or otherwise) of essential oils is based on reporting of adverse effects, although it can be difficult to confirm the validity of these reports, not least because other factors may play a part in producing an apparent adverse effect, whereas many true (direct) adverse reactions may go unreported. On the other hand, there are sufficient reports of the effects of some specific essential oils on humans to provide useful information and to warrant caution. Where these case reports relate to non-pregnant use, it is wise to consider the additional stress on an expectant mother and the fetus and to include the relevant oils in the list of essential oils contraindicated in pregnancy (see Chapter 4).

Caution must also be applied, however, to the nature of the evidence used to demonstrate benefits or hazards of essential oils. There is considerable research evidence on the risks of herbal medicines, but these cannot automatically be applied solely to essential oils, which are only one constituent of herbal remedies. Any proven risks of herbal preparations may be due either to another isolated ingredient or to a combination of chemical constituents which do not occur in essential oils.

Evidence of the therapeutic effects of essential oils

Essential oils are thought to have strong anti-infective properties and have variously been claimed to be antibacterial, antiviral, antifungal, analgesic and anti-inflammatory. They have also been said to be relaxing or stimulating, or to have effects on the gastrointestinal or immune systems. Evaluation of essential oils in reducing subjective symptoms such as pain and anxiety or stress tend to be based on the use of a blend of essential oils, often combined with massage, from which it is difficult to elucidate the true therapeutic agent. There is, however, considerable *in vitro* evidence for the anti-infective properties of many essential oils, although the studies do not always involve oils commonly used in clinical aromatherapy and many studies are from the food production industry or from veterinary medicine.

A summary of some recent studies relating to common pathogens and essential oils used in aromatherapy, found on the National Center for Complementary and Alternative Medicine (NCCAM) database, is outlined in Table 3.1.[1] These have been classified into animal, *in vitro* and clinical research and that which has been conducted by the pharmaceutical industry. Table 3.2 outlines some general clinical studies on the pain-relieving effects of aromatherapy and Table 3.3 gives details of research on the use of essential oils for relaxation and the relief of stress and anxiety. It is interesting to

---

1   www.ncbi.nlm.nih.gov/pubmed?&orig_db=PubMed&cmd_current= Limits&pmfilter_Subsets=Complementary%20Medicine

note that certain essential oils, especially lavender, feature in many of the studies – not necessarily because lavender is the most clinically effective, but perhaps because it is the most popular or commonly used oil in general aromatherapy practice. Finally, Table 3.4 provides more detailed abstracts on recent maternity-specific studies; apart from massage, any studies involving other therapeutic interventions with the essential oils, such as music, have been omitted.

Table 3.1 Summary of some recent research on anti-infective properties of essential oils

AUTHORS AND DATE	TITLE	CONCLUSIONS
Boukhatem *et al.* 2014	Lemon grass (*Cymbopogon citratus*) essential oil as potent anti-inflammatory and antifungal drugs	Lemongrass oil may have anti-inflammatory and antifungal activities (pharmaceutical research)
Carmen and Hancu 2014	Antimicrobial and antifungal activity of *Pelargonium roseum* essential oils	Geranium and associated oils may be effective against *pseudomona, E. coli, Staph. aureus, C. albicans* (pharmaceutical research)
Chin and Cordell 2013	The effect of tea tree oil (*Melaleuca alternifolia*) on wound healing using a dressing model	Tea tree may be effective in wound healing (clinical research)
Dagli *et al.* 2015	Essential oils, their therapeutic properties, and implication in dentistry: A review	Lavender, cinnamon, peppermint, clove, eucalyptus, lemon and tea tree oils may have anti-infective effects beneficial in dental surgery (clinical research)
de Campos Rasteiro *et al.* 2014	Essential oil of *Melaleuca alternifolia* for the treatment of oral candidiasis induced in an immunosuppressed mouse model	Tea tree oil may be effective in combatting oral candidiasis (animal study)
Karbach *et al.* 2015	Antimicrobial effect of Australian antibacterial essential oils as alternative to common antiseptic solutions against clinically relevant oral pathogens	Tea tree, lemongrass and eucalyptus oils may be better antimicrobial agents than oral antiseptics (clinical research)
Satyal, Shrestha and Setzer 2015	Composition and bioactivities of an (E)-β-farnesene chemotype of chamomile (*Matricaria chamomilla*) essential oil from Nepal	Chamomile shown to be effective against *Staph. aureus, E. coli, C. albicans* and other organisms (*in vitro* research)

Table 3.2 Summary of some recent clinical studies on analgesic effects of essential oils/aromatherapy

AUTHORS AND DATE	TITLE	CONCLUSIONS
Ayan *et al.* 2013	Investigating the effect of aromatherapy in patients with renal colic	Inhalation of rose oil in conjunction with intramuscular (IM) diclofenac effectively reduces pain in patients with renal colic
Bakhtshirin *et al.* 2015	The effect of aromatherapy massage with lavender oil on severity of primary dysmenorrhea in Arsanjan students	Lavender oil massage decreased primary dysmenorrhoea in female students
Heidari Gorji *et al.* 2015	The effectiveness of lavender essence on sternotomy related pain intensity after coronary artery bypass grafting	Inhalation of lavender oil reduced pain in post-operative cardiac patients
Ou *et al.* 2012	Pain relief assessment by aromatic essential oil massage on outpatients with primary dysmenorrhea: A randomised, double-blind clinical trial	Clary sage, jasmine and marjoram oils combined with massage reduced intensity and duration of menstrual pain in healthy volunteers
Ou *et al.* 2014	The effectiveness of essential oils for patients with neck pain: A randomised controlled study	Marjoram, black pepper, lavender and peppermint self-administered via massage eased neck pain in self-selected patients

Table 3.3 Summary of some recent clinical studies on relaxation/stress-relieving effects of essential oils/aromatherapy

AUTHORS AND DATE	TITLE	CONCLUSIONS
Bikmoradi *et al.* 2015	Effect of inhalation aromatherapy with lavender essential oil on stress and vital signs in patients undergoing coronary artery bypass surgery: A single-blinded randomized clinical trial	Inhalation of lavender oil reduced systolic blood pressure but did not reduce perception of mental stress in post-operative cardiac patients
Chen, Fang and Fang 2015	The effects of aromatherapy in relieving symptoms related to job stress among nurses	Lavender inhalation reduced workplace stress in nurses
Jafarzadeh, Arman and Pour 2013	Effect of aromatherapy with orange essential oil on salivary cortisol and pulse rate in children during dental treatment: A randomized controlled clinical trial	Orange oil inhaled by children undergoing dental treatment significantly reduced cortisol and pulse rates
Karadag *et al.* 2015	Effects of aromatherapy on sleep quality and anxiety of patients	Lavender essential oil increased quality of sleep and reduced anxiety in patients with coronary artery disease
Watanabe *et al.* 2015	Effects of bergamot (*Citrus bergamia* (Risso) Wright & Arn.) essential oil aromatherapy on mood states, parasympathetic nervous system activity, and salivary cortisol levels in 41 healthy females	Inhalation of bergamot oil reduces stress and associated physiological parameters in health volunteers

Table 3.4 Summary of some recent research studies on aromatherapy and massage in pregnancy and childbirth

AUTHORS AND DATE	TITLE	ABSTRACT
Chen and Chen 2015	Effects of lavender tea on fatigue, depression, and maternal-infant attachment in sleep-disturbed postnatal women	Randomised controlled study of 80 postnatal women in Taiwan, with difficulties in sleeping. They were given either lavender tea, which they were required to inhale and then consume, or regular postnatal care only. Initial effects showed less fatigue and depression in experimental group but this appeared to be short-lived.
Kaviani *et al.* 2014	Comparison of the effect of aromatherapy with *Jasminum officinale* and *Salvia officinale* on pain severity and labor outcome in nulliparous women	Randomised controlled group of 156 labouring primigravidae who received either clary sage oil or jasmine oil by inhalation or distilled water via a face mask. Pain perception and the duration of the first and second stages of labour in the clary sage group were significantly lower than in the jasmine or control groups. There were no statistically significant differences between groups in relation to labour outcomes or infant Apgar scores.
Keshavarz Afshar *et al.* 2015	Lavender fragrance essential oil and the quality of sleep in postpartum women	Randomised clinical trial of 158 postpartum women who received either lavender oil at night or a placebo. Aromatherapy received four times a week for eight weeks was found to significantly increase the sleep quality in the intervention group compared to the control group.

Kheirkhah *et al.* **2014**	Comparing the effects of aromatherapy with rose oils and warm foot bath on anxiety in the first stage of labor in nulliparous women.	Randomised controlled trial of 120 primigravidae in labour, receiving either rose oil by inhalation and foot bath, warm water footbath or standard midwifery care. Both experimental groups had less perceived anxiety than the control, but there was little difference between the rose oil/footbath group and the footbath only group.
Namazi *et al.* **2014b**	Effects of *citrus aurantium* (bitter orange) on the severity of first-stage labor pain	Randomised controlled trial of 126 primiparous women in labour who received either inhalation of bitter orange oil or a placebo, repeated at 30-minute intervals. The aromatherapy group was found to experience a significant reduction in their perception of pain during the first stage. Author's note: Bitter orange is contraindicated in maternity aromatherapy.
Olapour *et al.* **2013**	The effect of inhalation of aromatherapy blend containing lavender essential oil on Cesarean post-operative pain	Triple-blinded randomised controlled study of 60 women given either inhalation of lavender oil or placebo oil, or standard care following elective Caesarean. The lavender group had less pain at 4, 8 and 12 hours post-operatively and greater satisfaction with pain medication. The placebo group and control group used significantly more analgesia than the lavender group. Conclusion: Lavender oil may be effective in reducing pain relief after Caesarean but not in isolation.
Rashidi Fakari *et al.* **2015**	Effect of inhalation of aroma of geranium essence on anxiety and physiological parameters during first stage of labor in nulliparous women: A randomized clinical trial	Randomised controlled study of 100 primigravidae in Iran who were given either geranium oil or a placebo by inhalation. Anxiety scores and diastolic blood pressure were significantly reduced in the experimental group.

cont.

AUTHORS AND DATE	TITLE	ABSTRACT
Sibbritt *et al.* 2014	The self-prescribed use of aromatherapy oils by pregnant women	Cross-sectional questionnaire of 8200 women in Australia. 15.2% of women self-administered aromatherapy during pregnancy. They were more likely to use aromatherapy for allergies or hayfever or for a urinary tract infection. Conclusion: Large numbers of women are using aromatherapy in pregnancy; there is a need for more education of both women and professionals.
Smith *et al.* 2011	Aromatherapy for pain management in labour	Systematic review of randomised trials on aromatherapy for pain relief in labour. Two trials were scrutinised (535 women). There were no real statistically different results when comparing the control group with the aromatherapy group for pain management, secondary use of pain relief, neonatal admission to special care baby unit, length of labour and birth outcomes. Conclusion: More research is needed on aromatherapy for pain relief in labour.
Yavari Kia *et al.* 2014	The effect of lemon inhalation aromatherapy on nausea and vomiting of pregnancy: A double-blinded, randomized, controlled clinical trial	Randomised controlled trial of 100 women with nausea and vomiting, comparing the inhalation of lemon essential oil with a placebo. Conclusion: There was a statistically significant difference between the groups on the second and fourth day of the trial, indicating that lemon essential oil could be useful for gestational sickness.

Chapter 4

Safety of Aromatherapy in Pregnancy and Childbirth

This chapter includes discussion on:

- toxicity and side-effects of essential oils
- over-dose effects
- adverse skin reactions
- respiratory reactions
- essential oils and the eyes
- oral toxicity
- carcinogenicity and cytotoxicity
- teratogenicity, mutagenicity and fetotoxicity
- emmenagoguic and abortifacient essential oils
- essential oils which may affect uterine contractions
- effects on maternal blood pressure
- other medical and obstetric conditions
- essential oils and breastfeeding
- aromatherapy and the neonate
- effects of essential oils on midwives and other care providers
- contraindications and precautions to essential oil use in maternity care.

Introduction

Aromatherapy constitutes an element of herbal medicine. However, unlike herbal medicine which uses whole plants, in aromatherapy the essential oils are extracted and used in isolation from the other plant constituents (see Chapter 2). In clinical aromatherapy practice, these highly concentrated oils are blended together and administered with the aim of achieving a therapeutic effect in the client.

The issue of safety of aromatherapy in pregnancy and childbirth is of concern both to professionals and to expectant mothers. Unfortunately, any potential risks are not always recognised, because many people believe that aromatherapy simply involves the use of fragrant oils and relaxing massage. They do not realise that the oils contain chemicals which, once absorbed into the body, work in exactly the same way as pharmacological drugs. However, if a substance has the power to be beneficial, then it must, by inference, be potentially harmful if it is misused or abused – and it is this misuse which is so alarming in respect of pregnant women (and their babies).

Essential oils can be more hazardous, if used inappropriately, than some herbal remedies or teas, because the concentration of chemicals in the essential oils is so much more significant. Essential oils are also volatile and fat soluble, unlike water-soluble herbal remedies, and because they are lipophilic they can pass rapidly across membranes within the body, so any potential toxicity can be intensified beyond that seen with medicines produced from the whole plant (see Chapter 3 on pharmacokinetics). There is growing concern amongst aromatherapy producers, practitioners and researchers in relation to the increased general use of aromatherapy, since the incidence of sensitivities and adverse reactions has increased, particularly contact dermatitis and severe respiratory effects. In addition, the increase in use of other chemical substances, including perfumes, cleaning materials, incense sticks and aromatic candles, has added to the problem, making people generally more sensitive to all fragrances, while over-use of common essential oils has led to inadvertent abuse, with new sensitivities developing in susceptible people, although it is difficult to attribute these effects to specific chemical constituents. Repeated exposure to foods to which individuals are allergic (e.g. fish) can eventually lead to an anaphylactic reaction, and continual over-use of essential oils could eventually produce similar consequences.

All essential oils are toxic at high doses, especially if taken orally. Safe practice results from a comprehensive understanding of the science of aromatherapy (see Chapter 3) and an appreciation of how to minimise any possible adverse effects. This means not only having an understanding of essential oils and their use in general clinical practice, but also an ability to apply the principles of aromatherapy to its practice within maternity care. However, identification of precisely which essential oils are safe to use for childbearing women is still very much open to question. There is no definitive evidence that aromatherapy – or the individual essential oils – is safe during pregnancy. We make an assumption about *relative* safety, based on the absence of any real data and the fact that thousands of women have used aromatherapy oils prior to and during pregnancy without any apparent adverse effects – or at least without any formal reporting of adverse effects. Unlike drug preparation, there is no requirement to prove 'beyond reasonable doubt' that an essential oil is safe before it is made available to the market, partly because essential oils, unlike herbal remedies, are viewed as 'cosmetics'. In any case, it would be impossible to obtain ethical committee approval to conduct formal randomised controlled trials on the safety of essential oils in pregnancy. This then poses the 'chicken and egg' dilemma of whether or not specific essential oils, or the general practice of aromatherapy, should be investigated to demonstrate its effectiveness or whether we need evidence of safety in the first instance. There would be no point in having evidence of one without the other, since essential oils may be effective but then found to be unsafe, or vice versa. (See Chapter 3 for further discussion on aromatherapy research.)

Practitioners and expectant mothers attempting to elicit information about the safety of essential oils in pregnancy and birth will find a plethora of conflicting and confusing advice, particularly in books or on Internet sites aimed at the general public, which frequently contain misleading and sometimes potentially dangerous information. Aromatherapy textbooks, professional aromatherapy organisations and insurance companies providing practitioner indemnity cover usually err on the side of caution when considering pregnant clients, without any real foundation or supporting evidence. This is, perhaps, more to do with protecting the practitioners and their relevant organisations from the threat of claims against them for alleged obstetric negligence than about any firm understanding of how essential oils and aromatherapy can be applied to pregnancy and childbirth. Also, professional regulations and insurance criteria are devised for practitioners who are not midwives and who may, without further training, have a lay person's anxiety about working with pregnant clients. Further, even where there appears to be some evidence either supporting or refuting the safety of aromatherapy/essential oils in pregnancy, there may be other studies with conflicting results – and this can be confusing to all concerned.

It is wise, however, to set the issue of safety in context. We must remember that aromatic oils have been used for thousands of years by millions of people, many of whom will have been pregnant or breastfeeding. In the Western world we are exposed to essential oils every day of our lives, in perfumes, bath products, cosmetics, food flavourings, incense sticks, aromatic candles and other commercially produced substances. Conversely, the ready availability of essential oils in high street health stores or via the Internet, and the popular belief that aromatherapy is 'just' aromatic oils and massage, coupled with the origins of UK aromatherapy in the beauty therapy business, means that the issue of safety appears to have been dismissed by many consumers. This extends to ill-informed healthcare professionals whose use is often based on the same misconceptions as those of their clients and who fail to acknowledge the professional boundaries within which they should practise. (See Chapter 5 for more on professional accountability.)

Practitioners using aromatherapy for pregnant and labouring women must be aware of those essential oils which are contraindicated in general and those which should be avoided specifically during the preconception and antenatal periods, labour and the puerperium. They must also understand the reasons for these contraindications and precautions in order to justify their practice.

Toxicity and side-effects of essential oils

When considering potential risks associated with aromatherapy, there are some essential oils which are known to be toxic (poisonous) to humans, whereas others, which may be safe enough, can trigger sensitivities in susceptible individuals. The main factors that govern the safety of an essential oil for therapeutic administration revolve around the general contraindications, the known side-effects and its possible toxicity. Common side-effects, which can lead to toxic reactions if unrecognised, uncontrolled or mismanaged, include adverse skin reactions and general pharmacological effects on individual physiology. In terms of toxicity, two of the general issues are oral toxicity and carcinogenicity, while in maternity care, the concerns extend to possible teratogenicity and mutagenicity, oils which are potentially abortifacient or emmenagoguic and how the physiology of pregnancy and the pharmacology of the essential oils interact.

Certain essential oils are potentially toxic to humans and are therefore completely contraindicated in clinical aromatherapy. These oils are listed in Box 4.1. It will be noted that some of these named plants are also used to produce herbal or homeopathic remedies, which are prepared and used differently from essential oils, so care must be taken to ensure that the product used is appropriate, whether for general clients or for those who are pregnant. For example, arnica essential oil should not be used at all in clinical aromatherapy, whereas homeopathically prepared arnica, which is said to work energetically rather than pharmacologically (see Chapter 3), is well known as a suitable remedy for post-delivery perineal bruising. Some contraindicated essential oils have similar names to others which are acceptable in aromatherapy, such as the prohibited *bitter* almond, versus sweet almond, which is safe to use as a carrier oil (except for anyone specifically allergic to almonds). Others relate to the part of the plant from which the essential oil has been obtained, some parts being safer than others – for example, cinnamon *bark* should be avoided, but cinnamon oil (from the spice) can be used in general aromatherapy (but not pregnancy).

In addition to the totally contraindicated essential oils listed in Box 4.1, Tisserand and Young (2014) advise that a number of others should be avoided throughout pregnancy and during the period of breastfeeding. Although many of the listed oils are less well used in clinical aromatherapy than others, it is useful, for the sake of completeness, to identify them here – see Box 4.2. Many of these contraindicated essential oils come from plants and herbs in general use, such as dill, fennel, oregano, parsley and sage, and some women may ask about the culinary use of herbs during pregnancy. On the whole, the addition of small amounts of herbs in cooking is acceptable, since the amount of essential oil in a few sprigs of the plant will be minimal. However, herbal teas also contain essential oils, as well as other constituents which may possibly be harmful at this time, and women should be advised to drink herbal teas in moderation, generally keeping to no more than three cups a day. A few herbal teas should be avoided in pregnancy, including parsley, fennel and sage, all of which contain chemicals which may trigger uterine muscle spasm, possibly, in early pregnancy, leading to miscarriage.

Box 4.1 Hazardous essential oils contraindicated in clinical aromatherapy

Armoise (mugwort)	Elecampane
Arnica	Fennel, bitter
Basil, exotic	Horseradish
Birch, sweet	Mustard
Bitter almond	Origanum
Boldo leaf	Pennyroyal
Broom	Pine, dwarf
Buchu	Rue
Calamus	Sassafras
Camphor, brown or yellow	Savin
Cassia	Savory, summer
Chervil	Tansy
Cinnamon bark	Thuja
Clove, bud, leaf or stem	Vanilla
Costus	Wintergreen
Deertongue	Wormwood

Box 4.2 Additional essential oils which should be avoided during pregnancy and breastfeeding

Anise and star anise	Ho leaf
Black seed	Hyssop
Calamint	Lavender, Spanish
Carrot seed	(*Lavandula stoechas*)
Chaste tree	Myrtle
Cypress, blue (*Callitris*	Oregano
intratropic)	Parsley, leaf and seed
Dill seed	Sage
Fennel, sweet	Yarrow
Feverfew	

Adapted from Tisserand and Young (2014)

Over-dose effects

Where individuals are adversely affected by specific essential oils known to be safe for clinical aromatherapy, reactions most commonly relate to inappropriate dosages. This particularly applies to reproductive toxicity (Cragan *et al.* 2006) (see pages 105–110). The normal aromatherapy dose for a fit, healthy, non-pregnant adult is 3%. However, where it is deemed appropriate and safe enough to administer essential oils via the skin or respiratory tract for maternity clients, the dose should be kept to 1–1.5% (or even 0.5%) in pregnancy, while for labour and the puerperium a maximum dose of 2% can be used. (See Chapter 2 for information on calculating dosages.) Midwives and other professionals working with pregnant women must have an understanding of acceptable safe doses and ensure that their own practice follows currently acknowledged guidelines. Expectant mothers should be advised to take care when adding essential oils to the bath water at home – 4–6 drops, diluted in a small amount of carrier oil, is sufficient. Sadly, cases are known to this author in which women have so enjoyed the aromas that they believe (incorrectly) that adding more essential oil to the water is beneficial, sometimes to their detriment.

However, possible 'over-dosing' can occur even when the appropriate essential oil and correct dose have been selected, the development of reactions being related to the duration or frequency of use. Unfortunately, this is often seen in maternity care when pregnant or labouring women (or maternity professionals) unwittingly continue the use of aromatherapy beyond the period that is therapeutically justified. For example, women should be advised that vaporisers should be used for no more than 10–15 minutes at a time and certainly never left on all night as often happens. The nostrils can only absorb a certain number of molecules from the volatile essential oils. Prolonged use means that once the nostrils are saturated with molecules, continued exposure may lead to over-saturation, which results in side-effects.

Similarly, the frequency of use should be considered, with no single essential oil being used continuously for more than three weeks. This is easily avoided by alternating essential oils with similar therapeutic properties so that the balance of chemical constituents is slightly different. For example, if a client required regular use of essential oils, perhaps to aid sleep on a nightly basis, three oils with similar effects could be used in rotation, such as lavender, chamomile and ylang ylang, thus avoiding over-use or over-dependence on a single essential oil.

Common, but usually relatively minor side-effects which occur through over-dose include:

- headache

- nausea

- dizziness

- loss of concentration/lethargy

- skin irritation (see adverse skin reactions)

- respiratory difficulties (see respiratory reactions).

Side-effects can affect *anyone* who is in contact with the vapours (i.e. inhalation and smelling the aromas) of the essential oils, including the woman, her partner, relatives and caregivers. These symptoms commonly, although not exclusively, occur with essential oils which have heavy or cloying aromas, such as chamomile, jasmine, lavender or geranium. Indeed, migraine headaches may be triggered by a variety of fragrances, not just essential oils, via an effect on the same cerebral receptors as alcohol.

The quickest and most effective solution when any of these reactions occurs is to discontinue the aromatherapy treatment and remove the essential oils, ventilate the room and advise the woman to drink plenty of water. If the essential oils have been applied in a massage blend, it may also be wise to wash the area of the body which has been exposed to the oils to minimise the risk of continuing absorption.

The same applies to the midwife, doula or therapist who reacts to prolonged exposure or heavy use of essential oils. She should wash her hands, drink a glass of water and, if practical, extricate herself from the environment for a short period. Midwives must also be mindful of losing concentration, as this could adversely affect their ability to make clinical judgements in an emergency, or to drive when working in the community setting.

It is also important to ascertain whether the mother's symptoms are due to the essential oils, are related to the physiological effects of pregnancy or indicate the onset of pathological complications. For example, in the case of headache in late pregnancy, the practitioner needs to be able to differentiate whether a reported headache is a reaction to an aromatherapy treatment, or due to stress, tiredness, dehydration – or severe pre-eclampsia. Dizziness may be due to the effects of one or more essential oils, physiological or pathological changes in blood pressure or haematocrit, or associated with some other condition such as a severe infection. As a general rule, reactions to treatment will occur during or within 24 hours of the aromatherapy treatment, although development of any of these symptoms following treatment should not simply be disregarded as such. Symptoms occurring after the first 24 hours are unlikely to be due to the treatment, although again, the possibility should not be dismissed, particularly as some essential oils remain in the tissues for up to 72 hours (see Chapter 3).

Guidelines for avoiding over-dose of essential oils

Over-dose reactions occur from the use of inappropriate essential oils, dosages or method of administration, or from the prolonged or frequent use of essential oils generally considered safe. It is therefore important to adhere to the following guidelines:

- The maximum dose for blended essential oils should be 1.5% in pregnancy, 2% in labour and the puerperium.
- Vaporisers should be used for no more than 10–15 minutes at a time.
- Avoid using specific essential oils continuously (daily) for more than three weeks.
- Differentiation between reactions to essential oils, normal physiological effects of pregnancy or developing pathology is vital.
- Apply 'first aid' measures in the event of suspected over-dose.

Adverse skin reactions

There are two main types of reaction which can occur when essential oils are administered via the skin: contact dermatitis, and photosensitivity, although both types can be difficult to predict. Common essential oil constituents which cause skin issues include those containing high levels of the terpene limonene, as well as phenols including eucalyptol, geraniol and isoeugenol (contact dermatitis) and furanocoumarins, particularly bergapten (photosensitivity).

Allergic contact dermatitis can occur with certain essential oils in susceptible women, even when the blend is well diluted. Initial irritation from contact with essential oils leads to sensitisation, resulting in inflammation and the formation of antibodies in the local area. Very occasionally, the inflammatory process can disturb melanin and cause it to pass into the dermal layer of the skin, causing hyper-pigmentation, especially in dark-skinned people. Continued or repeated exposure to an essential oil acting as an allergen can cause an accumulation of antibodies, eventually triggering a more severe reaction, and possibly anaphylaxis. Lis-Balchin (2010) suggested that the general incidence of allergic contact dermatitis steadily rose in the 20 years prior to 2010. Allergic airborne contact dermatitis, with inhaled essential oils coming into contact with the nasal passages, has also been reported (Schaller and Korting 1995). These known increases may be due to greater usage of fragrances and essential oils, better reporting of side-effects, more scientific understanding of the risks, increased exposure to chemicals in all walks of life, or to some other, as yet unidentified, factor.

Traditionally, patch testing was used by many aromatherapists to determine whether an individual client was sensitive to specific essential oils. This involves the application of a single drop of the essential oil to the particularly sensitive skin on the underside of the upper arm, which is then covered with a plaster and left for 24 hours. Although this practice is no longer commonly used as a routine procedure, Corazza et al. (2014) advocate its use as a diagnostic technique when a skin reaction has actually developed. In any case, it would not be practical to undertake patch testing for pregnant and labouring clients, since it would require the woman to return to the clinic or treatment room 24 hours after her first appointment, which would be a waste of her time and the practitioner's. In addition, the dynamic nature of labour suggests that the essential oils used may change as the first stage progresses, and it is certainly to be hoped that the baby will have been born within 24 hours!

In maternity aromatherapy it is preferable to become familiar with the essential oils most likely to cause skin irritation and to identify those women who may be susceptible. The main culprits are essential oils from the *Compositae* plant family, such as chamomile (Paulsen, Christensen and Andersen 2008), although this is seen more commonly with German chamomile (*Chamomilla recutita*) than Roman chamomile (*Chamaemelum nobile*). There are also many reports in the literature of adverse reactions arising from chamomile tea, as opposed to the essential oil – primarily contact dermatitis (Anzai, Vázquez Herrera and Tosti 2015) but even anaphylactic shock has been documented (Andres et al. 2009). Contact dermatitis is also seen with tea tree oil (*Melaleuca alternifolia*) (Larson and Jacob 2012) and is particularly problematic when oxidised (Rutherford *et al.* 2007). Other oils implicated include peppermint (Herro and Jacob 2010) and eucalyptus (Gyldenløve, Menné and Thyssen 2014). In a study by Posadzki, Alotaibi and Ernst (2012), lavender, tea tree, peppermint and ylang ylang were the oils which most commonly caused adverse effects, with contact dermatitis being the primary issue.

Women with pre-existing skin conditions such as eczema and psoriasis, those with dry or itching skin and those who are allergic to specific plants such as chamomile, or to certain perfumes or other cosmetics, should avoid the relevant essential oils. Doses should be kept to the minimum required for a therapeutic response, and if there is any doubt, dermal administration of any essential oils should be avoided. The number of essential oils used in any blend should be limited to a maximum of three to allow for prompt identification of the offending oil. Also, essential oils should generally not be used neat on the skin, although there are a few exceptions to this rule – usually for very localised application over a small area, such as over a verrucca.

There is a greater risk of contact dermatitis amongst those providing aromatherapy than their clients, especially when the oils are administered via massage in which the repeated friction to the hands may compromise the skin further. Midwives, doulas and therapists with a tendency to skin reactions should take care to wash their own hands thoroughly after using any essential oils and may even need to avoid using certain oils in their practice. The question of whether gloves should be worn has been raised by some authorities in previous years. Whilst this may be wise during blending, especially if a large batch of blends is to be prepared, it would be neither practical nor pleasant, for the mother or the practitioner, for gloves to be worn for massage.

Photosensitivity, a reaction of the skin to a substance when exposed to ultraviolet light, is often quoted as a potential side-effect of essential oils. This is thought to occur mostly with the citrus oils such as bergamot, lemon, lime, grapefruit, sweet orange, etc., due to the presence of furanocoumarins, particularly bergapten. Bergamot, which is high in bergapten, is thought to be the main culprit, causing reddening and darkening of the skin in light-skinned people. Given that pregnant women have high levels of melanocytic hormone and are therefore prone to burning in direct sunlight, rather than tanning, it is wise to be cautious about the dosages of citrus oils, even though they are amongst the safest oils for use in pregnancy. Women with recent acquisition of a suntan should be treated with caution and it may be best to avoid bergamot and other oils which can potentially trigger photosensitivity.

Any theoretical risk of photosensitivity can be minimised by ensuring that the skin which is in contact with citrus essential oils is not then exposed directly to strong sunlight for a few hours – covering the skin will negate any potential effect of the ultraviolet light. The risk of photosensitivity is at its highest in the first two hours after dermal application, gradually decreasing over the following eight hours. Keeping doses to a minimum, as with contact dermatitis, will also help. Where a mother is wearing clothing which reveals significant areas of bare skin, the practitioner can either suggest a treatment avoiding these areas, or choose different essential oils. Women who are more susceptible to light sensitivity include those with very pale skin and eyes, typically the 'English rose' complexion, with those with red hair and green eyes, or many freckles, or women with vitiligo or albinism being most at risk. The potential for photosensitivity can be further reduced by using furanocoumarin-free (FCF) bergamot oil, distilled lemon or lime oils and mandarin, sweet orange and tangerine oils.

Guidelines for minimising adverse skin reactions from essential oils

- Take a history from the mother about her skin condition, any sensitivities and personal or family history of atopic dermatitis.
- Be aware of the essential oils most likely to cause adverse skin reactions or photosensitivity.
- Caution should be used with women with a history of eczema, psoriasis or other skin conditions: if necessary, avoid essential oils.
- Generally avoid the use of neat essential oils on the skin.
- Dilute essential oils to an appropriate proportion for the stage of pregnancy, labour, etc.
- Do not add undiluted oils to the bath water.
- Use the minimum dose necessary to achieve the desired therapeutic effect.
- Cover the skin for at least two hours after exposure to photosensitive essential oils or avoid direct sunlight.
- If in doubt, avoid dermal administration of essential oils altogether.
- In the event of severe adverse reactions, wash the area with water and unperfumed soap for at least ten minutes, expose the skin to the air to allow for evaporation of any remaining oil, and treat any skin rash with an appropriate barrier cream or antihistamine.

Respiratory reactions

During any aromatherapy treatment, essential oils evaporate and the volatile molecules are then inhaled, irrespective of the primary method of administration. The respiratory tract is very vascular and provides a large surface area for the essential oil metabolites to be absorbed. Fragrances and their chemical constituents are known to be respiratory irritants in some people, possibly causing bronchial and alveolar inflammation and exacerbating pre-existing conditions such as asthma, sinus congestion or hayfever. Long-term exposure to essential oils can be more problematic than occasional contact, and symptoms will be exacerbated by frequent or prolonged exposure, possibly affecting caregivers more than the pregnant and labouring women.

Two main types of reaction occur as a result of inhalation of essential oil molecules: adverse reaction to the chemical constituents or adverse reactions to the aromas. Occasionally, an essential oil will be pungent enough in some people to cause *sensory irritation*, activating the trigeminal or vagal nerves in the nose, mouth and eyes and causing tickling, stinging or burning sensations. Sensory irritation is non-allergic although it may exacerbate existing allergic conditions such as hayfever. Oxidised essential oils can also produce these symptoms of irritation in some people.

Bronchial hyper-reactivity, as occurs in conditions such as asthma and allergic rhinitis, is characterised by reflex bronchospasm, dyspnoea and air hunger, triggered, usually, by histaminic or cholinergic substances. Some essential oils may induce a psychosomatic adverse reaction to a particular fragrance in women with asthma or hayfever, due to an association with the aromas of plants which cause their condition to flare up, even though there are none of the usual allergens present in the oils.

A similar, though somewhat controversial condition, *sensory hyper-reactivity*, has no known aetiology but appears to be an allergic reaction specifically associated with the inhalation of fragrances. Women are thought to be 3–4 times more likely to be affected by sensitivity to aromas than men (Scheinman 1996). A case is known to this author of a midwife who inhaled clary sage essential oil for the first time, as she was unfamiliar with its aroma, and who had an immediate respiratory reaction which was severe enough to warrant a transfer to the Accident and Emergency department. This midwife is unable to use clary sage oil in her personal practice and needs to take care when entering rooms where the oil has recently been used by others.

Since it is difficult to predict who may respond in such a way, it is vital that midwives and other caregivers are aware of the possibility of adverse respiratory effects on their clients, themselves and others in contact with the oils. It is also difficult to determine which essential oils are most likely to cause respiratory reactions. In general, practitioners must be aware of the 'double dosing' which effectively takes place during a treatment, from both the primary method of administration, such as massage or adding oils to the bath *and* the inhalation of the aromas. Professionals should be mindful of the necessity to regulate the total amount and the choice of essential oils for any individual. Tisserand and Young (2014) advise keeping the percentage blend for massage in people with asthma or sensory hyper-reactivity to 1% or less to avoid over-exposure to vapours which may trigger an attack (this advice applies equally to practitioners and other people in the same room as the woman receiving aromatherapy).

If an adverse respiratory reaction occurs, the individual should be removed from the room, preferably to fresh air. If the condition continues, transfer to the emergency medicine department at the local hospital is advised. Anyone who has reacted adversely to a specific essential oil should not come into contact with that oil in the future and care should be taken regarding contact with any other essential oils, particularly those high in the same chemical constituents as were in the offending oil.

Guidelines for minimising respiratory reactions to essential oils

- Be alert to the potential for people to react adversely to chemicals or aromas when inhaled.
- Check the mother's medical history for respiratory disorders, sensitivity to perfumes, and tendency to allergic reactions in general.
- Alert others in the room to the use of oils, including partners, staff and visitors.
- Use the lowest possible dose for the required therapeutic effect.
- Use no more than 1% dosage for massage in those susceptible to reactions.

Essential oils and the eyes

On a general note, essential oils should be kept away from the eyes as they may cause corneal abrasion. Irritation of the eyes may also occur on inhalation of some essential oils, notably those containing pinene or limonene (monoterpenes). In the event of oils coming into direct contact with the eyes, they should be flushed thoroughly for at least 15 minutes with cool water; contact lenses should be removed after the first five minutes to avoid additional scratching.

Oral toxicity

Poisoning from accidental over-dose is the most frequently reported severe toxic reaction to essential oils in humans, occurring most commonly from ingestion of an undiluted essential oil, in amounts higher than those considered suitable for a therapeutic response. Generally, reported poisonings have involved essential oils which are not normally used in aromatherapy, such as wintergreen or wormseed oil, although death is rare. Tisserand and Young (2014) cite several accounts from the last hundred years in which other essential oils such as cinnamon, clove and camphor have caused poisoning. There have also been reports of oils such as eucalyptus and tea tree resulting in toxicity, particularly amongst children, in Australia and, more recently, in the United States. Ingestion of essential oils in amounts large enough to cause poisoning can result in contact excoriation to the mouth or lower in the digestive tract, as well as organ-specific complications from dispersion through the central circulation – for example, neurotoxicity, hepato- or renal toxicity, causing symptoms such as lethargy, slurring of speech, ataxia and muscle weakness.

Essential oils should rarely be administered by mouth in therapeutically effective doses. However, this rule must be balanced by the fact that they are commonly used in minimal amounts as flavourings in food products and are therefore ingested on a daily basis by most people. Essential oils should not be administered orally, even in therapeutic doses, to pregnant women.

It is vital to keep essential oils out of the reach of children, who may inadvertently drink the oil. In this event, medical help should be sought immediately and if possible, the local poisons advice centre should be contacted for specific advice. In the United Kingdom, members of the public and healthcare professionals needing emergency advice can telephone 111, the NHS Choices information line. Professionals working in direct clinical practice can also register with the UK National Poisons Information Service. In addition, the Medical and Healthcare Regulatory Authority (MHRA) operates a Yellow Card reporting system for adverse effects from drugs. This has recently been extended to include herbal and homeopathic medicines, although there is little direct provision for the reporting of adverse effects of essential oils.

If someone ingests any essential oils, it is vital to avoid inducing vomiting, as this may add to any mucus membrane irritation and excoriation and could cause aspiration into the lungs. The mouth should be rinsed well with water and the person transferred to hospital. However, if the person is unconscious or fitting, nothing should be given by mouth, and normal resuscitation measures should be employed before and during urgent transfer to hospital. The essential oil bottle should be taken with the attendants to enable rapid identification of potential chemicals responsible.

Carcinogenicity and cytotoxicity

Little information is available regarding the potential carcinogenic (abnormal or new cell growth) and cytotoxic (harmful to cells) effects of essential oils. Some of the oils recognised as being carcinogenic are contraindicated in clinical aromatherapy (e.g. camphor, sassafras and calamus) largely as a result of the high safrole content, which can cause hepatotoxicity, although adverse effects are not apparent at lower doses. The majority of research on this aspect of aromatherapy has been conducted through animal studies in which individual chemical constituents are tested, rather than whole essential oils. Examples include studies on α,β-thujone as found in sage and wormwood oils (National Toxicology Program 2011a), pulegone from pennyroyal (National Toxicology Program 2011b) and elemicin, a constituent of nutmeg oil (De Vincenzi, De Vincenzi and Silano 2004). In addition, trials involving rodents have generally required daily exposure to high doses of essential oils given orally for some considerable time (often many months) in order to induce neoplastic growth. This fact suggests that cautious use of essential oils considered safe in clinical practice, whether for pregnant clients or not, pose no real threat of cancer. Indeed, more work appears to be in progress to evaluate the *anti*carcinogenic (cytotoxic) potential of selected essential oils, such as frankincense (Ni *et al.* 2012) and tea tree (Ireland *et al.* 2012).

Teratogenicity, mutagenicity and fetotoxicity

Much has been written about the possible risks of essential oils causing embryonic malformations (teratogenicity) or developmental anomalies later in the pregnancy (mutagenicity). Some of the very small chemical molecules within the lipid-soluble essential oils cross the placental barrier from the mother via the nuclear membranes of the cells. These then gain access to the genes which produce the various proteins required to promote development of the fetal immune system, tissues and growth factors (transcription and translation). Although the significance of this process is not fully understood, it is thought that the metabolism may be helped by the presence of local enzymes. However, exposure of the fetus to any alien substances, including essential oils, could lead to genetic changes such as teratogenic or carcinogenic effects, making the individual more susceptible to illnesses such as cancer in later life. Major anatomical structural formation occurs in the embryo during the early weeks, but later exposure to essential oils may affect fetal physiological functions, different systems being sensitive to different chemical constituents at varying gestations. In addition, large fetal metabolites, which would normally be excreted back into the maternal circulation, may be unable to diffuse across the placental barrier because of the untoward presence of the essential oil molecules. These unfavourable metabolites may then also interfere with later development or fetal wellbeing, although the issue is largely theoretical.

Essential oils should not be administered via the mucus membranes (oral, vaginal or rectal administration) in pregnancy, as the levels of essential oil constituents reaching the fetus via the placenta will be excessively high.

Although essential oils administered dermally or by inhalation cross the placental barrier, the concentration reaching the fetus is much less than that in the mother. However, the blood–brain barrier is not well developed in the fetus, allowing substances such as essential oils to reach the CNS, which is susceptible to chemical damage and where the effects are likely to be more pronounced than on the maternal CNS. On the other hand, the relative immaturity of the fetal liver means that it is incapable of metabolising a compound into a more toxic one, unlike in an adult, thus giving the fetus a degree of protection from harmful or potentially harmful constituents in essential oils. Some essential oils administered to the mother will, in any case, be in very low concentrations once they reach the fetus, due to rapid detoxification by the maternal liver.

There has been very little research on the teratogenic or mutagenic effects of essential oils, and studies have, of necessity, been conducted on rodents given extremely high oral or intravenous doses. Despite this, the findings have been largely inconclusive. In addition, specific constituents have usually been tested in isolation, rather than as part of an essential oil, whereas in clinical aromatherapy these constituents work synergistically with all the other components, often reducing the impact of single constituents. Further, those essential oils which have been studied have largely involved oils not commonly used in clinical practice, and notably not those considered safe enough for use in maternity care. For example, Domaracký et al. (2007) investigated the effects of sage, thyme, cinnamon, oregano and clove bud oils on mice, none of which should be used in human pregnancy. While thyme had no effect on embryonic development, oregano and clove bud caused cell death, and cinnamon and sage reduced the number of nuclei and distribution of embryos. High concentrations of sweet fennel, also contraindicated in pregnancy, may be toxic to pregnant rats in high concentrations, but does not appear to have teratogenic effects (Ostad, Khakinegad and Sabzevari 2004).

Some essential oil constituents, in high enough concentrations to become toxic once passing through the placental barrier to the fetus, may have serious effects. Several cases of accidental ingestion of camphor oil by pregnant women have been reported over the years, and although most babies survived, the general toxicity of camphor precludes its use in pregnancy. Oils containing sabinyl acetate, found in several oils such as savin, wormwood, plecanthrus and Juniperus pfitzeriana, are considered to be amongst the most dangerous constituents for pregnant women, plecanthrus in particular being 'strongly teratogenic' (Tisserand and Young 2014). Methyl salicylate, found in wintergreen and sweet birch essential oils, which are not used in aromatherapy, may impair closure of the neural tube in pregnant rats (Overman and White 1983). Fetal neurotoxic effects have been shown with benzyl alcohol, a constituent found in essential oils such as benzoin. Although most cases appeared to be exposed to benzyl alcohol as a component of medications or cleaning agents, severe neonatal consequences of perinatal use have been recorded, including respiratory distress, neurological impairment and poor growth. Thujone, found in sage oil, as well as other oils not used in clinical aromatherapy, is also known to be neurotoxic to adults, although its effects on the fetus are less well documented. For a comprehensive discussion on the safety of essential oils in pregnancy, see Tisserand and Young (2014).

Emmenagoguic and abortifacient essential oils

There is no evidence to suggest that essential oils classed as emmenagoguic (promoting menstruation-like vaginal bleeding) are also abortifacient (causing miscarriage). Additionally, there is no justification for prohibiting the use of an essential oil in the first trimester under the misconception that it may cause miscarriage. Certainly, these same oils should not be viewed as a means of inducing labour, the physiology of which is different from that which involves cyclical shedding of the endometrium or spontaneous expulsion of the embryo/fetus. An essential oil is either (relatively) safe in pregnancy – or it is unsafe. Caution should be employed throughout the preconception, antenatal, intrapartum and postnatal periods with all essential oils.

The confusion about emmenagoguic essential oils and their potential to cause miscarriage appears to have arisen in Victorian England, when women seeking to terminate an unwanted pregnancy drank pennyroyal oil (*Mentha pulegium*, a member of the mint family). This oil is extremely hepatotoxic, nephrotoxic and neurotoxic, possibly due to the high levels of the ketone pulegone, and women who drank it frequently became severely ill or even died. Subsequent miscarriage was probably due to the inability of the ill woman to sustain the pregnancy, rather than to any direct abortifacient effect of the pulegone or any other chemical in the oil. Despite this, pennyroyal has long had a reputation as an abortifacient herb, notably when taken orally as a tea over several days. As a herbal remedy it is no longer considered safe for any therapeutic uses.

Unfortunately, the tradition of ingesting pennyroyal oil led to a decades-long misconception that essential oils high in ketones (see Chapter 3) will cause vaginal bleeding, leading to miscarriage, and many aromatherapy textbooks perpetuate this myth, for which there is no hard evidence. Over the years, numerous essential oils have been classified as 'abortifacient'. However, the justification for not using them during pregnancy is based on their general toxicity, which may affect the mother and/or cause fetal death, rather than causing the smooth muscles of the uterus to contract, thus leading to miscarriage. To complicate matters further, the abortifacient effects which may be attributed to specific plants do not always apply to the essential oils when isolated from those plants, since many other constituents of herbal medicines can produce similar reactions. Essential oils still used in some countries today to initiate miscarriage include parsley – its abortifacient effect is thought to be due to the apiole content, rue, although the pilocarpone considered responsible for making the uterus contract is not found in the essential oil – and plecanthrus, due to the presence of sabinyl acetate, which is toxic.

Essential oils which are commonly used in general clinical aromatherapy and which may be abortifacient or emmengagoguic include juniper berry, clary sage, jasmine and rose. Juniper berries, used in the production of gin, have long had a reputation for inducing abortion, although there is confusion between *Juniperus communis*, from which juniper essential oil is produced, and savin (*Juniperus sabina*), a contraindicated oil. On the other hand, in the respected German Commission E monographs on herbal medicines, juniper essential oil has been accused of having a nephrotoxic effect (Blumenthal, Goldberg and Brinckman 2000). It would therefore be wise to class juniper berry oil as a contraindicated oil for maternity clients, due to its effects on the renal system, until more robust evidence is available. Clary sage, jasmine and rose appear to be safe enough to use in labour and with caution in the puerperium although they should be avoided in pregnancy. These specific oils are discussed elsewhere (see Chapter 7).

Essential oils which may affect uterine contractions

Tisserand and Young (2014) cite studies as far back as 1913 and up to the present day in which essential oils have been found to reduce uterine contractions when tested on pregnant animals. They list 14 essential oils and numerous individual chemical constituents which may be responsible. Popular essential oils used in therapeutic aromatherapy practice which may inhibit contractions include tea tree (Lis-Balchin 1999), manuka and kanuka (Lis-Balchin, Hart and Deans 2000), as well as several oils contraindicated in pregnancy, such as thyme, black seed and caraway.

Interestingly, research also suggests an inhibitory effect of ginger, lavender, sweet fennel and the apparently abortifacient oils named above, as cited by Tisserand and Young (2014). These conflicting findings may arise from the effects of specific chemical constituents within the oils which, when used in certain doses, may reduce contractions. Conversely, different doses of the same oil may have the opposite effect and actually stimulate contractions; or the apparent abortifacient effect may be due to some other mechanism such as causing fetal death or placental separation rather than stimulation of the myometrium. In addition, some animal studies have been conducted on the smooth muscle of the ileum. Whilst one can then assume that any findings may apply also to the smooth muscle of the uterus, the difference in intrapartum action of the myometrium (contraction and retraction) and the complex hormonal physiology of pregnancy and labour may influence whether an essential oil reduces or accelerates uterine contractions.

It is difficult to state with any degree of certainty whether specific essential oils inhibit or augment contractions in human childbirth. Where studies have been conducted on labouring women, it is normally the *concept* of aromatherapy as a clinical modality rather than the use of specific essential oils which has been tested. Further, where midwives have administered aromatherapy, this has frequently been with a blend of several essential oils, often given in combination with massage. This then brings in another dimension, since the massage may be relaxing or analgesic, which will then indirectly promote labour progress through a reduction in cortisol and a corresponding rise in oxytocin. Some studies, such as that by Rashidi Fakari *et al.* (2015), use specific essential oils (in this case, geranium) in a massage blend, whereas others use different methods of administration, such as a warm water foot bath with rose oil, as in the study by Kheirkhah *et al.* (2014).

However, despite the variable formal evidence, one must not dismiss anecdotal evidence based on extensive clinical practice. Clary sage oil, in particular, is a cause for concern, given the widespread contemporary belief amongst pregnant women (and midwives and doulas) that it can trigger contractions. Clary sage essential oil was used to good effect during labour in the large longitudinal study undertaken by Burns *et al.* (2000), although it was used in conjunction with other oils. Unfortunately, it has now become known amongst pregnant women as a 'natural' means of inducing labour, thus potentially avoiding the necessity for medical induction, especially in post-dates pregnancy (see Chapter 6). The excessive and premature use of clary sage by women who do not understand the physiological processes of labour has resulted in numerous reports to this author of preterm labour, when used before 37 weeks gestation, and fetal distress and even stillbirth when used inappropriately or in excessively high doses immediately prior to and during labour at term. (See also Chapters 6 and 7.)

One must also take account of the progress of labour in any individual. Where labour is well established, no essential oils thought to enhance uterine action, particularly clary sage, should be used as this may lead to hypertonic contractions. Even if the contractions reduce in strength, length or frequency, it is important to address first the other factors which may be influencing this change, such as dehydration, pain, anxiety and fear, or obstructed labour. Women who are having labour artificially (i.e. medically) induced, either by prostin pessary, Propess™, syntocinon or membrane rupture, should refrain from using essential oils for at least an hour to allow the medical treatment to take effect. If subsequent doses of the drugs are given, a similar period without additional essential oils should be observed.

Guidelines for minimising adverse effects on uterine activity

- Be aware of those essential oils generally considered to be contraindicated in human pregnancy.
- Avoid essential oils which are high in ketones in the preconception and antenatal periods.
- Adhere to general guidelines on dosages in pregnancy and labour.
- Avoid essential oils in labour which may have an inhibitory effect on the myometrium (e.g. tea tree, manuka and kanuka).
- Avoid essential oil of rose until 34 weeks gestation, and clary sage and jasmine until term.
- Employ extreme caution with clary sage in labour – consider it as 'nature's syntocinon'.
- Attend to other physiological reasons when contractions appear to have slowed down in labour before resorting to clary sage.
- Advise women to avoid teas made from parsley, sage and fennel during pregnancy.

Effects on maternal blood pressure

Traditionally, several essential oils, including thyme, rosemary, sage, wormwood and hyssop, have been identified as being *hypertensive*, which probably originates from the work of Valnet in the mid-1960s. It will be noted that wormwood is completely contraindicated in clinical aromatherapy, while the others should not be used in pregnancy. Some aromatherapy textbooks state that rosemary is safe enough in the third trimester, although the 1.8 cineole and camphor content of rosemary suggests otherwise (Tadtong *et al.* 2015). Rosemary has been shown to have an 'antihypotensive' effect (i.e. theoretically hypertensive) in a study by Fernández *et al.* (2014) on surgical patients with low blood pressure. Some essential oils appear to have an indirect hypertensive effect, which is part of the complex mechanism related to convulsions induced by excessively high doses of the oils, when given orally, this evidence being based on animal studies. On the other hand, individual chemical constituents, such as methyl salicylate, may give rise to poisoning (toxicity), which in turn leads to hypertension or convulsions. Methyl salicylate is found in several essential oils not used in clinical aromatherapy, but also in ylang ylang in very small amounts. However, evidence suggests that ylang ylang is an extremely relaxing oil which actually has the effect of lowering cortisol levels and thus, indirectly, lowering the blood pressure rather than raising it (Hongratanaworakit and Buchbauer 2006; Kim *et al.*

2012). This may be due to the synergistic effect of the other constituents in ylang ylang essential oil.

Some essential oils and their chemical constituents have been shown to have *hypotensive* effects, such as 1.8 cineole (Moon *et al.* 2014), which is found in eucalyptus. However, caution should be applied here, given that some studies are conducted on animals given large doses orally or intravenously, whilst many human studies involve administration via the skin. Massage in itself has a relaxing and vasodilatory effect which lowers the blood pressure, or the mechanism may be related to the alteration in other parameters such as anxiety (Rashidi Fakari *et al.* 2015). As with all issues related to toxicity, there is a difference in effect dependent on whether the essential oil is ingested, inhaled or applied to the skin. Olfactory stimulation alone may elicit different physiological responses as shown in relation to grapefruit and lavender oils by Nagai *et al.* (2014). Lavender oil (*Lavandula angustifolia*) appears to have a particularly valuable role in reducing systolic blood pressure (Bikmoradi *et al.* 2015), possibly due to a reduction in cortisol (Hongratanaworakit 2011; Kim *et al.* 2012).

Whilst there is no real evidence for effects on the blood pressure from specific essential oils when used appropriately and in normal doses, caution should be taken with women with diagnosed fluctuations in blood pressure, either hypertension or hypotension. Blood pressure in pregnancy follows a recognised physiological pattern: it tends to be similar to the pre-pregnancy levels during the first trimester, then falls during the second trimester due to the vasodilatation induced by increased progesterone, despite an increase in fluid volume. During the third trimester, the blood pressure returns to normal levels or may increase; a diastolic of 90 mm Hg, or more than 20 mm Hg, on the booking blood pressure is considered high. After delivery, the pressure gradually returns to normal levels, although any woman who has suffered severe (fulminating) pre-eclampsia is at greater risk of severe hypertension causing eclamptic fits in the first 48 hours of the puerperium.

The range of essential oils covered in this book does not include any which are considered to be directly hypertensive. Maternity professionals should administer all aromatherapy treatments with caution in women with hypotension. In practice, it is more likely that massage or the relaxation effects of some essential oils will contribute to lowering the blood pressure, but care should be taken to avoid postural hypotension when the mother gets up after a massage treatment, especially in the second trimester. Given that lavender and ylang ylang have been shown to have a hypotensive action, these should also be avoided when a mother has an epidural anaesthetic *in situ* because of the similar effects of bupivacaine. Clary sage oil is also thought to reduce the blood pressure but is contraindicated until term. If a labouring mother who has received clary sage to stimulate contractions later chooses to have an epidural, the clary sage should be discontinued.

However, the issue of using aromatherapy in pregnancy and labour is more significant in women with *hyper*tension as their condition is already compromised and there may be very real risks to both mother and baby. Whilst women with mild to moderate hypertension may benefit from a relaxing aromatherapy treatment, care must be taken with any mother on antihypertensive medication, to avoid potentiating the effects of the drugs, either from a physiological or pharmacological perspective. Women exhibiting signs of fulminating pre-eclampsia should not receive aromatherapy at all, by any means, including vaporisation.

Guidelines for minimising adverse effects on maternal blood pressure

- Avoid all essential oils considered to have a hypertensive action, as well as those containing large amounts of methyl salicylate.
- Be aware of physiological variations in blood pressure in individual women.
- Avoid lavender, ylang ylang and clary sage in labour if the mother has an epidural anaesthetic.
- Women on antihypertensive medication should not receive essential oils considered to be actively hypotensive (i.e. lavender, clary sage and ylang ylang).

Other medical and obstetric conditions

It is wise to be extremely cautious when using essential oils on pregnant women with pre-existing medical conditions. The mother's condition is compromised by being pregnant, with a risk of complications arising in relation to a medical condition, or to the progress of the pregnancy, to fetal development (possibly as a result of medications) and to the overall maternal and fetal wellbeing. These women require close medical supervision, and to introduce a therapy which is not yet well regarded by many conventional medical practitioners, and for which there is limited access to conclusive research evidence on safety, especially during pregnancy, is not good practice. Health professionals must be able to justify their actions and it would be extremely difficult to do so with any real authority in the case of pre-existing medical conditions or obstetric complications. Women on any medication are at risk of interactions between the drugs and the essential oils, either from potentiation or inhibition, and the liver will need to work harder to detoxify both substances.

However, the level of caution exercised by professionals providing maternity aromatherapy will be dependent on the degree of severity of the mother's condition. There are some conditions which may be complete contraindications to aromatherapy and others which would be considered precautions. The decision to treat with essential oils may also relate to the environment in which the practitioner is working (e.g. in sole, independent practice versus a main maternity unit which has the necessary emergency facilities in case of complications arising), the parameters of local clinical guidelines (see Chapter 5) and whether or not the mother is admitted to hospital as an in-patient. Obviously, the more serious her condition, the less appropriate it may be to provide aromatherapy treatments. The conditions covered below need particular consideration:

Epilepsy is a *complete contraindication* to aromatherapy in pregnancy. Non-pregnant people with epilepsy can develop unexpected and individual reactions to essential oils, although those whose condition is well controlled by medication should normally be no more at risk than non-epileptic people. However, pregnancy can cause the epilepsy to become unstable, especially if a change of medication is required. Not only is the condition itself compromised by the pregnancy, but maternal and fetal wellbeing will be compromised by the epilepsy. Conversely, certain essential oils have the potential to cause convulsions in any person, including when administered via the skin. Of the essential oils commonly used in clinical practice, rosemary and sage, as well as some types of lavender (spike lavender or *Lavandula stoechas*) may be potentially toxic to the CNS, which suggests that they should not be used in pregnancy, birth or the puerperium for any woman, irrespective of the manifestation of epilepsy.

Another absolute contraindication is *major cardiac disease*, which normally worsens considerably during pregnancy because of the extra fluid volume and pressure on the cardiovascular system. If a mother is an in-patient due to the interaction between the cardiac condition and the pregnancy, no aromatherapy treatment should be given. In those with minor cardiac conditions, such as a heart murmur, essential oils rich in menthol (e.g. peppermint and spearmint) should be avoided as these are thought to be cardiac stimulants which may cause dysrhythmias.

Vaginal bleeding is always a cause for concern during pregnancy. Any woman who is threatening to miscarry should not use essential oils (or receive massage while there is active blood loss). In the case of antepartum haemorrhage, no aromatherapy treatments should be given at all until bleeding has stopped, and only then if the mother's condition is such that there is no continuing risk, either to her or to her baby. Placenta praevia grades 3 or 4 may be considered contraindications to aromatherapy, especially in the third trimester, whereas grades 1 and 2 may be precautions. Clary sage appears to have some effect on smooth muscle (see earlier) and has been known to cause excessively heavy lochia in the puerperium. Therefore it is recommended that clary sage is avoided in women with retained products of conception, to prevent the possibility of torrential secondary postpartum haemorrhage.

Pregnant women with *coagulation disorders*, or needing anticoagulant medication such as warfarin, should not receive aromatherapy. This does not preclude them from enjoying a massage treatment, subject to normal precautions employed in the event of thrombo-embolic disorders. Tisserand and Young (2014) list several essential oils which could affect either coagulation or platelet aggregation, although their advice to avoid these oils refers mainly to oral use. However, they do suggest that breastfeeding women – and presumably all mothers in the early puerperium discharging lochia – should avoid ingestion of those essential oils which have anticoagulant properties. Interestingly, their list includes sweet fennel, an essential oil especially beneficial for promoting lactation, although dermal administration does not seem to be a problem.

Women with pathological *anaemia* (as opposed to physiological hydraemia) should be treated with caution. There is no substantive evidence that essential oils affect red blood cells, although recent studies, mainly on oils not generally used in aromatherapy practice, suggest that some constituents may cause destruction of erythrocytes. However, any woman with the genetic disease glucose-6-phosphate dehydrogenase deficiency (G6PD) should avoid mint oils such as peppermint and spearmint, due to the abnormal breakdown of erythrocytes which occurs as part of the condition.

Some constituents of essential oils could be potentially toxic, but are rapidly detoxified by the liver. This suggests that women with *liver or gall bladder disease*, including cholestasis, or hepatic compromise, such as alcohol-related disease, should not use essential oils. Tisserand and Young (2014) suggest that certain types of eucalyptus and peppermint should be used with caution in those with non-gestational cholestasis, but again this refers to oral administration. Women with severe renal disease should also generally avoid aromatherapy in pregnancy. This is because the glomerular filtration system and fluid balance mechanisms will be compromised, and because of the higher risk of toxicity to the kidneys from essential oils, even in low doses. However, most recorded cases of nephrotoxicity are related to oral over-dose, commonly with essential oils which are contraindicated in clinical aromatherapy.

Women with pre-existing or gestational *diabetes mellitus* may receive aromatherapy but should be treated with care, dependent on the stability of their condition. Essential oils which may affect blood sugar, causing either hypo- or hyperglycaemia, when taken in large oral doses include geranium, lemongrass, sweet fennel and certain types of basil, marjoram, tea tree and thyme (Tisserand and Young 2014). Since the mechanism of action is not fully understood, caution should be used when providing aromatherapy for any pregnant woman with diabetes. If insulin is required to regulate the blood sugar, it may be wise to avoid using essential oils completely and to offer only massage with a carrier oil.

Aromatherapy is contraindicated in those who suffer *migraines* since this condition is associated with an increase in sensitivity to aromas, and the use of aromatic oils could possibly precipitate an attack. Any *pyrexia* or *infective condition* is also a contraindication to aromatherapy, not least because the treatment itself may cause a rise in temperature, but also because the woman is likely to feel too unwell to receive treatment. In addition, certain oils (e.g. black pepper) are known to have rubefacient properties – in other words, they cause reddening and warming of the skin when applied topically, which could exacerbate cutaneous effects, including the temperature and the rate of absorption of essential oils. Some essential oils, such as sweet fennel, anise and myrtle, contain high levels of anethole, which is thought to be oestrogenic. Therefore women with breast or other *oestrogen-dependent tumours* should avoid these oils. However, as any pregnant woman with cancer will be under close medical scrutiny and may be on medication, treatment with essential oils should be avoided, although gentle massage with a carrier oil only may be welcomed.

Offering aromatherapy treatment to pregnant women with some obstetric conditions also needs careful consideration. This is not due to any real risk of essential oil constituents having an adverse effect, but more to do with the issues discussed earlier – already compromised wellbeing and the fact that these women will be under medical supervision. For example, *multiple pregnancy* is not, of itself, a reason to refrain from using aromatherapy, and, indeed, many women expecting twins may appreciate the relief of some of the pressure symptoms which are so much worse than in women with a singleton pregnancy. However, in the case of a higher multiple pregnancy (triplets or above), it is recommended that treatment is only provided by midwives who are already experienced in using aromatherapy in pregnancy, and possibly only provided in an environment where extra vigilance can be employed to prevent the mother having any untoward reactions to treatment. Similarly, abnormal fetal presentation or lie (*breech presentation, transverse or unstable lie*) would be considered a precaution, although this is more in relation to massage than to specific essential oils. The same applies to severe *polyhydramnios* or *oligohydramnios*, especially when known to be related to a fetal malformation.

Women in active *preterm labour* should not be treated with essential oils, even those thought to inhibit uterine action such as tea tree (Lis-Balchin 1999; Lis-Balchin *et al.* 2000). However, once contractions have ceased, gentle treatments with a low percentage blend of fairly mild oils, such as the citrus oils, may be given. As mentioned, several cases of inadvertent preterm labour as a result of inappropriate use of essential oils such as clary sage, or herbal remedies including raspberry leaf tea, have been reported to this author, and midwives are advised to enquire of the mother whether she may have taken any natural remedy which could have contributed to the onset of premature contractions. This will need to be tackled diplomatically as the mother may be reluctant to provide information, but questions will also need to be incisive as some women may not realise that they have taken any natural remedies – for example, if they have been drinking herbal teas for enjoyment rather than for a particular effect.

Any *fetal condition* should also serve as a warning about the appropriateness of aromatherapy. Where there are *reduced fetal movements* or *intrauterine growth retardation*, this may be considered a contraindication, but if it is deemed acceptable to provide aromatherapy, doses of essential oils should be kept to an absolute minimum – possibly 0.5%. Treatments should be of short duration and the choice of essential oils should exclude any about which there is any concern at all.

Guidelines related to medical and obstetric complications

- Be aware of conditions in which aromatherapy is completely contraindicated.

- Use professional discretion when working with women with conditions which constitute precautions to aromatherapy.

- If in doubt, avoid using essential oils – it may be possible to use carrier oil only for a massage.

- Adhere closely to maternity unit clinical guidelines as a protection for both the mother and the professional (see Chapter 5).

Essential oils and breastfeeding

Essential oils, like drugs, pass from the maternal circulation to the breastmilk. This is thought to be by a process of passive diffusion which can be influenced by protein binding, fat solubility and molecular size. Although the levels reaching the neonate will be considerably less than those in the mother, the baby must then metabolise the chemicals. If the mother is taking medication which could have severe side-effects on the neonate, breastfeeding may be contraindicated. However, if the drugs are safe enough to permit breastfeeding, caution may be necessary in the use of essential oils on the mother since the baby will then have additional chemicals to metabolise. Tisserand and Young (2014) advocate caution with several essential oils when a woman is breastfeeding. They include basil, lemon balm, lemongrass, myrtle and thyme, although most of these are contraindicated in maternity care for other reasons. Of interest is their assertion that tea tree should be avoided when breastfeeding due to the presence of citral, notably in the lemon-scented type.

Aromatherapy and the neonate

Essential oils should *never* be used on or near neonates and infants under the age of three months. There are several reasons for this:

- The baby's skin, which acts as a barrier to infection, does not mature for several months and is more sensitive and more permeable to essential oils, which may predispose the child to skin allergies in later life. Preterm infants are particularly vulnerable and essential oils should *never* be used in the special or intensive care baby unit.

- The neonate is less able to deal with any side-effects which may occur, particularly skin irritation from dermal application.

- The mother–infant relationship ('bonding') is partially dependent on smell recognition by the baby, which could be overwhelmed by the introduction of aromatic fragrances such as essential oils, especially those with strong aromas or when used in high doses.

- Bronchial or sensory hyper-reactivity may occur from the inhalation of essential oil vapours, as suggested by Wyllie and Alexander (1994) and Crandon and Thompson (2006). This applies to the inhalation of essential oils from room vaporisers, steam inhalation in the bathroom and direct dermal application of essential oils, as well as to commercial products containing essential oils or their constituents such as Olbas™ oil.

- The baby's immune system continues to mature after birth. Given that all essential oils have, to a greater or lesser degree, anti-infective properties, mainly against bacteria, but also viruses, fungi and other microbes, their use could slow down the maturation and development of the neonatal immune system, with the potential for lifelong difficulties in fighting infection.

Aromatherapy treatments for the mother should be carried out in a room away from the baby, although there seems to be little risk to the baby of being in contact with the mother once she has had an aromatherapy treatment. If the mother has had a full body aromatherapy treatment or used essential oils in the bath, the breasts should be washed with water before feeding the baby. Mothers should be advised that if they use essential oils in the bath at home, the baby should not be in the bathroom with them, in order to avoid them inhaling excessive essential oil molecules from the steam. Vaporisers should *never* be used in the baby's room.

Effects of essential oils on midwives and other care providers

Aromatherapy has an impact on those providing the treatment, as well as on any relatives of the client who may be present. It is important that midwives and other caregivers take care to protect themselves from the possibility of adverse effects. In conventional medical terms this can be likened to the need to protect oneself from diagnostic techniques such as X-rays. The risks to practitioners cannot be over-emphasised, especially when an individual is exposed to essential oils via inhalation or dermal absorption over a prolonged period of time (e.g. a full shift).

A midwife or other professional providing aromatherapy who is pregnant, breastfeeding or attempting to conceive, or who is undergoing fertility treatment, should avoid inhalation or direct contact with any essential oils contraindicated in pregnancy. Anyone who is epileptic, has a major medical condition or is taking medication which could be influenced by the effects of essential oils should take extreme care when caring for women using aromatherapy. If a caregiver experiences an adverse effect of any kind from professional use of aromatherapy, s/he should avoid using the relevant essential oils. These issues mean that clients' choices of essential oils will need to be limited to those which are safe for the practitioner.

Certain essential oils are thought to have effects which may not be revealed in pregnant clients – for example, clary sage, which was traditionally used in wines in the 17th century as a means of increasing the effects of the alcohol, may cause more rapid inebriation in a professional who has used the oil for a woman in labour and who then goes for an after-work drink in the pub. Clary sage can also stimulate a heavier than normal blood loss in menstruating women.

There are reports in the literature of aromatherapists being adversely affected by the oil which they use in their practice, including hand dermatitis (Crawford *et al.* 2004). Several anecdotal accounts have also been reported to this author, such as irritation of the eyes or nose, nausea, headache and menorrhagia.

Guidelines for protection of professionals using essential oils

- Practitioners who are pregnant, trying to conceive or undergoing fertility treatment should avoid using essential oils which are contraindicated in pregnancy.

- Midwives, doulas and therapists must be aware of the effects of all essential oils which they may use in their practice and take steps to protect themselves, their colleagues and visitors.

- Caregivers must be given the option to decline to use specific essential oils if they experience adverse reactions to them.

Contraindications and precautions to essential oil use in maternity care

Table 4.1 provides a summary of the contraindications and precautions outlined in this chapter.

Table 4.1 Contraindications and precautions to essential oil use in maternity care

CONTRAINDICATIONS	PRECAUTION
Epilepsy – absolute	Mild cardiac compromise (e.g. heart murmur)
Major cardiac disease	
Liver or gall bladder disease, cholestasis	Previous hepatic or biliary condition
Severe renal disease	Urinary tract infection, current
Pre-existing or gestational insulin-dependent diabetes mellitus	Non-insulin-dependent diabetes mellitus
Pathological anaemia	Previous low haemoglobin or other blood deficiency (e.g. folic acid)
Thrombo-embolic or coagulation disorders	History of previous thrombo-embolic disorders
Mothers on anticoagulants or drugs for similar disorders	Mothers on medication for other medical problems
Infectious conditions or unexplained pyrexia	Minor respiratory disorders, allergic rhinitis, sensitivity to fragrances
	Skin allergies, eczema, psoriasis, verrucas, etc.

cont.

CONTRAINDICATIONS	PRECAUTION
Severe asthma or major respiratory disorder	Twin pregnancy
Major skin conditions	Placenta praevia, grades 1 or 2
Multiple pregnancy – higher multiples	History of vaginal bleeding
Placenta praevia, grades 3 or 4	Labile blood pressure, diastolic of 85–90 mm Hg
Current vaginal bleeding	Severe hypotension, tendency to fainting, postural hypotension
Hypertension, with diastolic above 90 mm Hg; fulminating pre-eclampsia	Breech presentation, transverse or unstable lie
Severe polyhydramnios or oligohydramnios related to severe fetal or maternal condition	Reduced fetal movements
Severe intrauterine growth retardation	History of preterm labour in this or a previous pregnancy
Preterm labour of unknown origin (current)	Booked for elective Caesarean
	Within the first hour following medical or surgical induction or augmentation of labour
	Epidural *in situ* in labour
	Excessive or malodorous lochia in puerperium
	Professional uncertainty

Chapter 5

Implementing Aromatherapy in Midwifery Practice

This chapter includes discussion on:

- education and training of practitioners providing maternity aromatherapy
- implementing aromatherapy: aims and outcomes of the intended service
- logistical issues to be considered
- health and safety issues
- writing a business proposal
- financial considerations
- professional accountability
- *Standards for Medicines Management*
- supervision of midwifery practice in relation to aromatherapy
- escalating concerns
- indemnity insurance cover
- clinical guidelines
- evaluating the maternity aromatherapy service.

Introduction

The process of implementing any new strategy into midwifery practice can be difficult and frustrating. Once midwives have decided what service they wish to provide and why, they must then deal with the process of change management. When introducing aromatherapy, it is essential for midwives to work within 'the system' and not to be so overtaken with enthusiasm that problems are encountered because they have attempted to rush the process. Setting up a working group to develop the aromatherapy service can be helpful, providing a forum for discussion and a means of allocating the work to be done amongst several people, as well as offering mutual support when things are going slowly or difficulties arise.

Although many maternity units are keen to establish a general aromatherapy service, midwives must remember that their first priority is to the women and babies in their care. Aromatherapy is not a conventional aspect of midwifery practice and care must be taken not to deviate from the primary objective of care provision. Midwives are qualified to practise *midwifery* and must justify their reasons for bringing in a new strategy which is outside the mainstream provision of maternity care.

It is often easier to consider implementing this new initiative as a means of minimising or resolving problems which present issues for management, such as the need to reduce costs, intervention or litigation risk, or to improve maternal satisfaction. For example, offering aromatherapy as an alternative to medical induction of labour for women with post-dates pregnancy could reduce induction rates, costs of oxytocics and other drugs associated with the 'cascade of intervention' arising from induction of labour. Using aromatherapy in this way could also help to relax women sufficiently to enable their bodies to work more effectively through a rise in oxytocin, making it more likely that labour will start spontaneously. Aromatherapy and massage fit particularly well with the desire to offer additional means of pain relief in labour, and the return to a more nurturing way of caring for women can often bring other, unanticipated but positive results, such as increased recruitment and retention of midwives (Burns *et al.* 2000).

There are, however, several aspects of the change management process which need to be considered before aromatherapy can be introduced into midwifery practice.

Education and training of practitioners providing maternity aromatherapy

Clause 13.5 of the Nursing and Midwifery Council (NMC) *Code* (NMC 2015) requires midwives to complete any necessary training before carrying out a new role. Maternity-related aromatherapy should involve an in-depth study of *both* clinical specialities, and any professional using essential oils for pregnant, labouring or newly birthed mothers must have a thorough understanding of all aspects of care. Midwives and doulas need to concentrate on learning about the principles of aromatherapy, including relevant physiology, chemistry and pharmacology, as well as how to blend and administer the oils safely and appropriately. Conversely, aromatherapists will need to study reproductive anatomy and physiology, and develop an appreciation of the conventional maternity services and their own roles and responsibilities when caring for maternity clients, whilst also applying their existing knowledge of aromatherapy to its use for maternity clients.

The extent to which an individual practitioner studies each element will depend on their professional background and their knowledge and experience to date. For example, midwives will already have an understanding of pregnancy-related anatomy and physiology and will be working within the maternity services; doulas working as the mother's advocate may have a good understanding of the psycho-emotional aspects of childbirth and may perhaps be more in tune with the concept of holism and energetic medicine. Aromatherapists will obviously have a working knowledge of how, why and where essential oils work but may not understand the intricacies of orthodox antenatal, intrapartum and postnatal care or the specific issues relating to safety in pregnancy.

All practitioners must acknowledge the boundaries of their practice, dependent on their existing qualifications, experience and insurance. Above all, the safety of expectant mothers and their babies is paramount. Table 5.1 gives a summary of the *minimum* requirements for education and training of any professional intending to offer aromatherapy to pregnant, labouring and newly birthed mothers.

Table 5.1 Education and training requirements for maternity aromatherapy practice

MATERNITY-RELATED CONTENT	AROMATHERAPY-RELATED CONTENT
Anatomy and physiology of pregnancy, labour and puerperium	Philosophy of complementary medicine
Possible pathology, recognition and actions, including emergency aid	Anatomy and physiology of skin, sense of touch, olfaction, respiration
Knowledge of contemporary antenatal, intrapartum and postnatal care	Pharmacology and pharmacokinetics of essential oils
Psychology of childbirth and basic listening skills	Basic chemical concepts, specific chemistry of essential and carrier oils
Health promotion and concepts of health	Therapeutic properties of essential oils and related research
Appreciation of healthcare ethics, legal aspects and professional accountability	Methods of administration
Understanding of research methodologies, application of research findings to clinical practice	Methods of blending
Understanding of role of midwives, doctors, other maternity professionals	Indications, contraindications and precautions to use of aromatherapy in pregnancy, labour and postnatal period

Within any maternity unit it is essential that all those using aromatherapy comply with the criteria laid down in the local clinical guidelines. Therefore, any midwife who is also a qualified aromatherapist should be required to undertake the same training course as other colleagues to ensure standardisation of practice and to facilitate audit of the service and treatments. It may also be appropriate for any new members of staff to complete the in-house course, even if they have used aromatherapy elsewhere, to ensure conformity. Midwives who have undertaken appropriate training in the use of maternity aromatherapy must support their colleagues' and students' learning to assist them in developing professional competence and confidence prior to permitting them to contribute to the aromatherapy service (*Code* clause 9.4) (NMC 2015).

Continuing professional development (CPD) is also essential in order to keep up to date with developments (*Code* clause 6.2) (NMC 2015) both in maternity care and in aromatherapy. Midwives must keep both their knowledge and skills up to date by taking part in appropriate and regular learning and professional development activities which assist in maintaining and developing competence and enhancing performance (*Code* clause 22.3) (NMC 2015). Aromatherapy updating, specifically applied to midwifery, should preferably be undertaken annually. This does not necessarily mean attending additional study days on aromatherapy; indeed, it is the application to midwifery/maternity care which is most significant and with which practitioners must maintain their competence and confidence.

CPD activities could include reading research studies, journals or new textbooks, visiting other maternity units in which aromatherapy is provided by midwives, writing up reflective case studies, including those with both positive and less positive outcomes, publishing an interesting case study in a professional journal, establishing a journal club in the local unit, developing a new profile for a specific essential oil to add to the available selection or recording conversations about aromatherapy which the practitioner has had with pregnant women.

The NMC requires registrants to undergo a process of revalidation, which is intended to strengthen registration renewal and is a continuous process concerned with promoting safe, effective, professional practice. All of the above suggested activities enable the midwife to comply with revalidation requirements, and could also be undertaken by other professionals as a means of maintaining contemporary maternity-aromatherapy practice.

The issue of midwives *cascade training* their colleagues in aromatherapy is a contentious subject. Many maternity managers supporting midwives to set up an aromatherapy service see fit to pay for just one or two midwives to undertake short training courses with external organisations, with the intention that these few midwives should then train the rest of the staff. However, midwives who have completed an initial course on aromatherapy are not sufficiently competent to pass on their knowledge to others without consolidating their own learning and gaining further experience in treating women during pregnancy, labour and the postnatal period, with the full range of essential oils in which they have been trained. For example, recognising possible side-effects associated with specific essential oils cannot be taught to others without substantial experience of using aromatherapy for this client group. Further, these midwives are not qualified aromatherapists and have therefore studied a limited amount of a subject which is totally new to them, unlike undertaking professional development directly related to midwifery, such as water birth workshops or courses on examination of the newborn. Not only do midwives need to be knowledgeable and competent to use aromatherapy, they must be able to apply the principles to midwifery practice, within the boundaries set by the Nursing and Midwifery Council (even when a midwife is a qualified aromatherapist).

In educational terms, learners are thought to retain about 60% of what they have been taught. Cascade training will therefore cause a natural dilution of the content imparted to others, with the worrying possibility that vital safety details may be missed, either by the trainers or by the learners. Cascade training should really only be considered by midwives with at least two years' experience of using aromatherapy in their practice, and preferably following involvement in the implementation process, including the development of local clinical guidelines.

In some maternity units, it may be possible for support workers or maternity care assistants to be involved in providing massage for women. However, the midwife must remain accountable for the treatment and should only permit junior colleagues to use aromatherapy oil blends if they have received training relevant to their scope of practice and competence (*Code* clause 11.1) (NMC 2015). The midwife is legally responsible for 'prescribing' the essential oil blend, so support workers are permitted to use only oils which have been blended by an appropriately trained midwife who has personally assessed the mother first, or oils which are commercially pre-blended, in order to perform massage. The midwife must ensure that the support worker fully understands the instructions and must confirm that the treatment given is appropriate and of the required standard (*Code* clause 11.3) (NMC 2015). Similarly, since student midwives are not legally accountable for the care of women during pregnancy and labour, any use of aromatherapy by a student must be under the direction of an appropriately trained midwife.

Implementing aromatherapy: aims and outcomes of the intended service

It is important to identify realistically the purpose of the intended aromatherapy service and the justification for its introduction in midwifery practice. Midwives should explore the immediate and long-term aims and goals and decide what could be achieved by offering aromatherapy to women in their care. The initial reason may be that it is an additional means of pain relief in labour, but longer-term outcomes might be a desire to minimise intervention, to reduce women's complaints, or to set up a research study. It can sometimes be easier to tackle implementation through formal research channels, but this does, of course, risk discontinuation of the service in the event of results which are not sufficiently statistically significant to justify aromatherapy use.

It is useful to undertake some preliminary research, both from the available professional literature and in practice. A literature search will reveal some of the contemporary evidence for safety and effectiveness of aromatherapy in pregnancy and/or labour. A feasibility study can be done, to assess women's interest in having an aromatherapy service (evaluating demand to justify implementation). It can also be useful to conduct a survey of midwifery and medical colleagues to ascertain their knowledge of and views on aromatherapy and their thoughts on the possible introduction of the service. Making contact with midwives in other units in which aromatherapy is already established can provide useful anecdotal evidence and also maintain morale – knowing that others have succeeded despite initial 'teething problems' can be reassuring and encourage midwives to continue with their proposal. Some midwifery or medical colleagues may be sceptical about complementary therapies, either because they know very little about the subject or have had negative personal or professional experiences. It is essential to present a convincing case which demonstrates that effective, safe and cost-effective aromatherapy services can be offered, based on both direct and indirect evidence.

One common objection raised by managers may be the lack of time and human resources to take on any new initiatives, and certainly there is a need to justify something such as aromatherapy, which is rarely seen as a priority. This is why it may be easiest to start by offering intrapartum aromatherapy since most women receive one-to-one care in labour, and aromatherapy treatments can be performed around observations, record-keeping and other clinical interventions. Simple massage techniques can also be taught to the woman's birth companion in a very short time, possibly leaving the partner to use the aromatherapy oils which the midwife has blended. Highlighting the beneficial effects of both massage and the essential oils, notably the fall in cortisol, which facilitates oxytocin release, may help to convince colleagues that intrapartum aromatherapy can contribute to reduced intervention through greater relaxation of women.

It is vital to be aware of any potential adverse effects (see Chapter 4), not least because obstetricians and midwifery managers are likely to raise this issue. Being alert to possible risks enables midwives involved in setting up the aromatherapy service to take steps in advance to minimise them and to demonstrate that the new service will be safe. It is useful to consider as many issues as possible before moving ahead with plans to bring in the aromatherapy service.

A SWOT analysis is one way of identifying some of the issues and helping midwives to focus on appropriate planning and implementation where the best chances of success lie. A SWOT analysis enables planners to identify **S**trengths, **W**eaknesses, **O**pportunities and **T**hreats (see Box 5.1).

Box 5.1 SWOT analysis for implementing aromatherapy in midwifery practice

Strengths

Compile a list of the aromatherapy and massage skills and strengths within the local team. What relevant resources, other than clinical aromatherapy skills, are there in the implementation team? Do team members have any experience of introducing new initiatives, developing guidelines, or overcoming obstacles in other areas of midwifery practice? This needs to be realistic as it demonstrates why a manager, supervisor or obstetrician should support the aromatherapy service.

How can the strengths within the implementation team be 'sold' to other colleagues, especially those who are sceptical? For example, would it be acceptable to offer mini-taster sessions of massage and aromatherapy so that colleagues who have not previously experienced aromatherapy have the chance to do so, perhaps from a hand or foot massage?

Weaknesses

It is also important to identify areas for improvement within the implementation team, including not only aromatherapy and massage skills, knowledge and application to midwifery practice, but also managerial and organisational skills and experience.

Where there are weaknesses or gaps in the expertise required, identify whether these can be improved, perhaps with further training, or whether there are other colleagues who may be able to fill these gaps.

Also pinpoint anything that should be avoided when setting up the aromatherapy service, such as extending it too far, too fast or inappropriately.

Opportunities

Establishing a new venture, whether it is aromatherapy or another service, can also create opportunities for mothers and for staff, individually and collectively, and it can be useful to determine these. Explore whether new opportunities might arise from changes in technology, local, national and international health policies and directives, or socio-economic and lifestyle factors. Could there be increased opportunities for the future of the aromatherapy service by building on the strengths within the implementation team and eliminating or reducing any weaknesses?

Threats

Identify any obstacles which may impact on the implementation process and maintenance of the aromatherapy service. For example, could any weaknesses in the team have an adverse effect on the possible success of the venture, and how could these problems be overcome? Identifying the threats can clarify what has to be done, but will also help to put matters into perspective.

Logistical issues to be considered

It is necessary to determine who is going to provide the aromatherapy service. It may not be appropriate for all midwives in the maternity unit to train in the use of essential oils and massage. A core team of designated aromatherapy-midwives could set up the initial service although this may risk the midwifery workforce becoming divisive – those who provide aromatherapy and those who do not ('them and us'). Also, if the number of midwives using aromatherapy is limited, how can equity of the service for the mothers be assured? It may, for example, be appropriate to limit the service to the birth centre and/or to home births, at least when it is first introduced. Will aromatherapy be offered as part of routine care for all women, or for all those who are low-risk?

Are any conflicts of interest likely to arise – for example, in the event of providing an antenatal clinic aromatherapy service, could there be problems in staffing it if the unit is busy elsewhere? Will midwives actually be allocated time to train in aromatherapy and to develop the service or will they be expected to do the work in their own time? This can occur in some units where management pays 'lip service' to bringing in a new initiative which may be popular with women but is not deemed essential to normal care nor, allegedly, financially viable.

Implementing aromatherapy is as much about examining current midwifery practice as it is about introducing something new. It does not have to take up an excessive amount of extra time, although initially more time will be needed to enable midwives to develop their competence and confidence. It is unlikely that the service will be available 24 hours a day, and women may need to be informed that the aromatherapy option is subject to availability, in the same way as for epidural anaesthesia or water birth.

It is wise to consider any factors which can influence the planning process and for the implementation team to be able to rationalise any limitations in provision of the service. For example, a comprehensive relaxation aromatherapy service cannot realistically be provided for all eligible women in a large maternity unit, and this may lead to devising a service which attends to specifically identified client groups – for example, women with a post-dates pregnancy, those in the latent phase of labour, those requesting additional methods of pain relief or perhaps a defined group such as teenagers or those with a previous poor obstetric history who may be extremely anxious.

Midwives should investigate where they are able to provide the aromatherapy service, taking into account the effects of aromas, chemicals in the oils and the women passing through the area. In the delivery suite it is wise to keep one or two labour rooms *completely* aromatherapy-free so that high-risk women and those with complex needs who may not be eligible to receive essential oils are not exposed to the aromas unnecessarily. An example of this is to avoid putting a woman admitted in preterm labour into a labour room in which contraction-promoting essential oils such as clary sage have recently been used.

If aromatherapy is offered in a ward setting, perhaps in the postnatal ward, what factors could interfere with service provision? Interruptions such as visitors, ward rounds, workload and simply the noise of a busy ward may all impact on the effectiveness of the aromatherapy treatments. If aromatherapy is available only for designated women, how practical is it to treat a postnatal mother at her bedside, to avoid upsetting those women who are not eligible to receive treatment, or adversely affecting those who should avoid it for medical reasons? Indeed, in the postnatal ward area, a separate room may be required in order to offer aromatherapy to women away from their babies, who should not, in any case, be exposed to the essential oil vapours.

Community midwives have an advantage in being able to use aromatherapy when caring for women having home births. However, it is necessary to decide how midwives will transport and store the oils, avoiding problems such as oxidation from oils which have been left in the car on a hot day, as well as considering the security of the oils.

Health and safety issues

In the United Kingdom, health and safety law states that employers must provide a safe working environment, relevant trained staff and written health and safety policies. Employers must also ensure there are no health risks to clients or employed and self-employed staff. All equipment used in the workplace must be fit for purpose, in good repair and regularly maintained, with written service records kept and correctly used by trained staff.

Electrical equipment must be checked annually by a qualified electrician, removed from use if faulty, sent for repair and accompanied by written records which are readily available for inspection. This includes any electrical vaporisers/diffusers used by midwives in their administration of essential oils, although for clinical safety, the practice of vaporising oils via diffusers should be avoided (see Chapter 4).

Manual handling regulations relate to ergonomics when lifting or moving equipment or clients, to reduce risks of injury. They require staff to learn safe practices for moving and handling, to take 'reasonable care' to ensure the safety of oneself and others and to use appropriate equipment to lift heavy loads. Midwives will be familiar with manual handling regulations because they are constantly at risk when facilitating births with women in a variety of positions. This understanding should be extended to ensuring protection of one's posture when performing massage on women, especially during the intrapartum period when women may be leaning over a birthing ball or in some position other than sitting in a chair or lying on a bed or couch.

The Control of Substances Hazardous to Health (COSHH) 1989 regulations relate to the use of chemical substances which may be harmful, toxic, corrosive or flammable. Employers and employees must be aware of potentially dangerous substances and health risks, including essential oils. Midwives should be familiar with local procedures for dealing with spillages of essential oils or in the event of an accident, such as a mother inadvertently drinking the oils, and must comply with local regulations designed to minimize accident risks. Essential oils must be handled and stored correctly and safely, ensuring that all substances, including pre-blended oils, are correctly labelled. Oils which are out of date must be disposed of in such a way that there is no environmental damage: it is permissible to dispose of unused or out-of-date essential oils and oil blends down the sluice or lavatory. Every step must be taken to ensure that there is no danger to mothers and babies, visitors and staff, both in terms of chemical and logistical safety (see Chapter 4) and complying with other legal requirements.

Writing a business proposal

Midwives will usually be required to present a business proposal to budget holders before any new initiative can be implemented. This does not have to be a lengthy process and, in fact, is more likely to be considered by managers if it is concise yet comprehensive. A business plan can be an extensive document, but a short plan of no more than two pages which summarises the proposal should be sufficient, although appendices of more detailed information may also be requested by the budget holders/decision-makers. A business plan should be structured, logical, realistic and appropriate to the service into which the new initiative is intended to be introduced. It should constitute a tool which contributes towards more detailed planning and is in keeping with the way the unit works. Box 5.2 presents a summary of possible aspects to be included.

Box 5.2 Writing a business proposal for the implementation of aromatherapy

Vision
Identify the service intended to be implemented – be specific, perhaps by relating to the intended aims such as reducing inductions of labour.

For whom will the aromatherapy service be provided?

Where and when will it be provided?

What is the time frame between proposal and implementation?

Mission statement
This should be short, memorable and focused.

For whom is the service intended and what are the benefits to individuals and to the maternity service as a whole?

Objectives
What are the intended/expected short- and long-term outcomes of the aromatherapy service?

How will outcomes be measured – for example, reductions in intervention, increase in normal births, reduction in drug use, improvement in maternal satisfaction scores, audit and evaluation of the service by midwives and mothers, etc.?

Strategies
Action plan:

- How will the aromatherapy service be set up?
- What needs to be done in order to establish it, by whom and by when?
- Practical and logistical planning.
- Development and approval of clinical guidelines.
- Appropriate means of record-keeping and audit.
- Training of staff.
- Purchasing and storage of oils.
- Budgeting and cost implications.

Financial considerations

When devising the business proposal it is essential to include a section on the financial issues. Midwives should identify the costs of setting up the service, including training, development time, cost of oils and any essential equipment, as well as any additional time needed to administer the service, and to evaluate and audit it. The source of funding required should be determined, including some discussion on alternative sources of funding if there are insufficient resources to set up and maintain the service. It may also be appropriate at this stage to consider whether the service will be free to women, or if there will be a charge for some parts of it.

The cost of implementing aromatherapy does not, in fact, have to be prohibitive. Training is likely to be the highest cost, but if this is budgeted over three years, the overall annual costs will balance out. An example of possible costs is included in Box 5.3, although some liberty has been taken in terms of time costs, as this will depend on the average hourly rate for the grades of the midwives involved.

The estimate is based on introducing an *intrapartum-only* aromatherapy service in a maternity unit with 6000 births annually. It assumes that one-third of the women will not be eligible on medical grounds, or will not wish to have aromatherapy or will progress too quickly to be able to take advantage of the service. For those 4000 women who could potentially receive aromatherapy in labour, the calculations are based on using 15 ml of grapeseed carrier oil in divided doses during the first stage.

It will be seen that the aromatherapy service in a large maternity unit can be implemented and run for an average annual cost of under £3000, including initial training and development. After the first three years, the annual cost would be less, despite the need for some continuing professional development. The difference in cost between a normal birth and a Caesarean section is approximately £1000 (NHS Institute for Innovation and Improvement 2013). It therefore stands to reason that using aromatherapy to achieve a reduction of three Caesareans per year would allow the unit to break even, without even accounting for the financial sequelae of Caesarean sections, such as admission of the baby to the special care unit, longer postnatal hospital stay, the possibility of a Caesarean in a subsequent pregnancy and the long-term urogenital complications that may occur, requiring medical care in the future. This can also be balanced against greater maternal satisfaction.

Box 5.3 Possible costs of implementing aromatherapy in a maternity unit (2016)

Training costs for 24 midwives, based on a three-day in-house course (equates to £187.50 per person)	£4500
Implementation and planning at the start of the project, including development of local guidelines, based on a working group of four midwives having four meetings of two hours each @ £20 per hour	£640
Cost of carrier oil, based on 4000 women x 15 ml grapeseed per person @ 60 litres per year x three years = 180 litres @ £55 per 5-litre bottle = 36 bottles @ £55	£1980
Selection of 10 essential oils for three years @ £350 per year	£1050
Total cost for aromatherapy service for three years	**£8170**
Total cost per year, for the first three years of the service	£2723

Professional accountability

The NMC gives tacit approval to the use of aromatherapy and other complementary therapies within the registrant's area of practice, on condition that the practitioner is adequately and appropriately trained to do so. Several of the NMC's documents give guidance which can be related to the use of aromatherapy in midwifery.

The NMC *Code* (NMC 2015) sets out standards of practice which midwives (and nurses) are required to meet in their obligations to the general public. Whilst *The Code* is a broad document designed to be applied to all areas of practice, its application to the use of complementary therapies within midwifery is implicit, although midwives may need help to draw this out from the general principles.

Women have the right to use aromatherapy oils during pregnancy, birth and early motherhood. The midwife must work in partnership with any woman who wishes to self-administer oils, acting as her advocate wherever possible (*Code* clause 2.1) (NMC 2015). More specifically in relation to aromatherapy, good practice involves facilitating the mother to choose which oils she prefers and not simply choosing those which are most clinically appropriate. If the mother does not like the aroma of a specific essential oil or a blend selected for its therapeutic purpose, she is unlikely to enjoy the treatment. This is one of the reasons why, in maternity units where pre-blended oils are used, there should always be an alternative option – for example, if a 'pain -relieving' blend is used for labour, a second blend should be available to enable women to choose the one they prefer.

The requirement to work in partnership applies equally if the mother prefers not to receive aromatherapy where it is offered by midwives. It is easy for midwives to become so enthusiastic about the benefits of aromatherapy that they may forget that some women could have objections to receiving treatment. They may dislike the aromas, may not want to be touched, as with massage, or may have particular moral, religious or spiritual concerns about what can sometimes be perceived as 'new age' therapies. The NMC (*Code* clause 4.1) (NMC 2015) reminds us to balance the need to act in the best interests of the woman, and that she has a right to accept or decline treatment.

Informed consent is crucial to all midwifery care (*Code* clause 4.2) (NMC 2015). Midwives offering aromatherapy must include not only information about the benefits of the proposed treatment, of both the essential oils and the method of administration, but also the potential risks and side-effects which may be experienced (see Chapter 4). The fact that verbal or written consent has been given should be documented, either on a specific aromatherapy record, or in the main maternity notes.

Any information given to the mother must be based on currently available contemporary evidence (*Code* clause 6.1) (NMC 2015). It is a common argument that complementary therapies 'lack evidence'. Whilst it is true that further research is required in order to build the evidence base for aromatherapy in general, and specifically in relation to maternity care, there is some anecdotal evidence which can be used to support maternity aromatherapy. In the absence of pure research findings, midwives must ensure that they work within contemporary boundaries for the use of aromatherapy, according to up-to-date textbooks, review papers and the principles of experienced authorities in the field of midwifery-aromatherapy. Examples of this would be the generally held principles that essential oils should not be added directly to the birthing pool water, nor vaporised in an institutional setting. If midwives choose to work outside these boundaries they *must* be able to justify their actions fully, if necessary in a court of law. If there are differences of opinion on the safe use of aromatherapy, midwives must discuss these and engage in informed debate (*Code* clause 9.3) (NMC 2015). As more evidence of safety becomes available, these practice principles may change, but until such time as more research is conducted, midwives should adhere to authoritative discourse on the safe use of aromatherapy in pregnancy and childbirth.

Essential oils can affect others who are in the room where aromatherapy is being used, including the midwife, the mother's partner and children and other staff (see Chapter 4), through inhalation of the vapours (aromas) or by direct skin-to-skin contact. The NMC's *Code* clause 19 (NMC 2015) requires midwives to be aware of, and to reduce as far as possible, the potential for harm associated with aromatherapy, by ensuring that everyone in contact with the oils is aware of this, keeping to the minimum dose required, avoiding aromatherapy use in public areas and monitoring practice of all those using it. It is not acceptable, for example, for diffusers to be left on the midwives' station or for strong vapours from one birth room to be noticeable in the corridor or other parts of the department.

The Code clause 13.4 (NMC 2015) emphasises the need to take account of one's personal safety whilst clause 4.4 raises the issue of conscientious objection and the need to arrange for a suitably qualified colleague to take over responsibility for the woman's care. This is a difficult issue, since it again relates largely to the effects of the essential oils on the midwife. There is an ethical issue around confidentiality if the midwife has a medical indication for avoiding contact with certain essential oils – for example, if she is pregnant and is unable to use oils which are thought to enhance uterine action in labour, such as clary sage. It may be that the midwife does not wish colleagues and managers to know about her pregnancy yet, but she must avoid exposing herself to the aromas of these oils. It should therefore be permitted in this situation, *without question*, for her to decline to use specific essential oils in her practice, although this may mean, on occasion, that she is unable to take over the care of a labouring woman who has been using those oils.

Midwives must maintain contemporaneous records on the use of aromatherapy (*Code* clause 10) (NMC 2015), including any advice which is given in the course of normal antenatal, intrapartum or postnatal care. As with all records, aromatherapy notes must be accurate, comprehensive and kept with the mother's normal maternity notes for the 25-year period required by law. A decision will need to be made about where aromatherapy records will be maintained – for example, by writing contemporaneous notes in the main pregnancy/labour record or devising a separate aromatherapy record sheet. Records should be included in the mother's hand-held notes and, where indicated, in the central maternity notes. In labour, if continuous electronic fetal monitoring is being used, it should be noted on the cardiotocograph (CTG) record when aromatherapy treatment commences and ends (even if the oils are administered by inhalation – for example, on a tissue). Computerised records should also include space for appropriate information to be recorded – for example if aromatherapy was used in labour for pain relief. Box 5.4 highlights the details which should be recorded for each aromatherapy treatment/administration, with an exemplar.

Women who are provided with a blend of essential oils for use at home, either during pregnancy or the puerperium, must receive the first treatment in the presence of the midwife. They must also be given written information about how to use the blend and what precautions they should take. The information leaflet should state:

- the indication for the blend
- what the blend contains (essential and carrier oils), including the percentage
- how to use it (method of administration)
- how much to use and how frequently
- what to do in the case of any queries or worries – information on possible minor side-effects
- after-care advice
- general safety information (e.g. 'keep out of reach of children', 'do not take by mouth', etc.).

Box 5.4 Recording aromatherapy treatments

Principle	*Example*
Indication for use of the essential oils and base oil; short- and longer-term goals	1. Pain relief in labour 2. To facilitate normal uterine action
Justification for the choice of specific essential oils and base oil; common and Latin names; relevant properties of the chosen oils	Black pepper (*Piper nigrum*) for pain relief; grapefruit (*Citrus paradisi*) and sweet orange (*Citrus sinensis*) for relaxation, to enhance mood and to balance aromatic blend Grapeseed carrier oil used as standard
Percentage of blend; number of drops of essential oil and amount of base oil used	2% blend: 10 ml carrier oil with 1 drop black pepper, 1 drop sweet orange and 2 drops grapefruit

Method of administration; if applied via massage, type of massage and areas of body; duration and frequency of treatment	Seated back massage for 15 minutes, stopping during contractions at mother's request; basic massage strokes taught to partner to continue treatment as required
	General antenatal relaxation treatment via back massage, as per local clinical guidelines
After-care advice given to the mother; any blended essential oils given for home use, appropriately labelled	Labour observations normal following massage: blood pressure, fetal heart normal; contractions maintained at 3:10
	Advised to drink water, avoid stimulants (e.g. coffee), rest, note any untoward symptoms, telephone triage if worried (antenatal treatment)
Evaluation of each treatment – mother's subjective evaluation and your professional objective assessment	Mother reported feeling more relaxed and better able to cope with pain; appeared to enjoy the massage and coping better with contractions

Standards for Medicines Management

The *Standards for Medicines Management* document (NMC 2010) directly refers to 'complementary and alternative therapies', and contains several more general statements that should also be applied to the pharmacological nature of aromatherapy essential oils. As with any pharmacological substance, essential oils should only be administered to the person for whom they are intended. A 'prescription' based on determining the most appropriate oils for the individual, administered in the correct dosage and frequency, via the correct method is vital to safe practice. Informed consent and comprehensive record-keeping are paramount, as noted above. Bottles of oils must be labelled correctly, with the names of the essential and carrier oils, percentage blend and expiry date. Since patient group directives (PGDs) generally refer to licensed medicines, these are not appropriate for aromatherapy and it may be acceptable to use the traditional 'standing order' approach for guidelines on the use of essential oils. Doctors, of course, cannot be responsible for prescribing or signing for aromatherapy, which is almost universally outside their qualifications.

Before discussing midwives' responsibilities when using aromatherapy in their own practice, it is useful to consider the issue of women using their own essential oils in pregnancy and especially in labour. Standard 5 (NMC 2010) refers to patients' own medicines including complementary therapies and herbal preparations (such as essential oils). The midwife should ask to see the oils and determine whether or not they are suitable for the mother to use. This can be difficult if the midwife has no knowledge of the remedies/ oils, but it is important to act as the mother's advocate and to support her in her wishes where at all possible. It is also necessary to explain to the mother how and why they will or will not be used – for example, she may be asked to discontinue using the oils in the event of deviations from normal progress. Women should also be strongly discouraged from offering their aromatherapy oils to other women. A record should be made of the woman's self-administration of aromatherapy, and ongoing assessment of her condition should be made to ensure that it is appropriate for her to continue to use the oils. It is not appropriate for women who are in-patients, particularly in the antenatal ward area, to keep essential oils with them in their bedside lockers, and if a woman is found to be in possession of essential oils she should diplomatically be requested to allow the oils to be locked away safely in the drugs refrigerator.

If midwives are using aromatherapy in their own practice, Standard 8 (NMC 2010) requires them to check that the woman is not allergic to the substance to be administered (in this case, essential oils). Midwives must also assess the individual and determine whether the essential oils are necessary and appropriate for the mother's condition (Standard 18.1), ensuring that they are compatible with any other medications the mother may be receiving (Standard 18.3) (NMC 2010). All essential oils, including those belonging to the mother, must be securely stored (Standard 18.4) (NMC 2010).

It is also a requirement that midwives keep to the laws of the country in which they are practising (Standard 20.4) (NMC 2010). Within aromatherapy, this particularly applies to the EU Directives on herbal medicines (see Chapter 2).

Supervision of midwifery practice in relation to aromatherapy

Adequate monitoring and supervision of the use of aromatherapy within midwifery practice is vital. Monitoring of individuals' practice and of the overall aromatherapy service should be undertaken by a senior midwifery colleague with appropriate aromatherapy knowledge and experience to help those using essential oils and massage, understanding the issues which arise and answering their questions, or referring them to alternative sources of information in the event that s/he is unable to answer them.

Currently, this is a rather *ad hoc* process, with Heads of Midwifery, other senior managers and consultant midwives often leaving it to the midwives who have implemented the service, assuming, probably correctly, that the 'shop-floor' midwives know somewhat more than the senior staff. However, it is not sufficient for midwives who have learned the minimum in order to implement this new 'tool' of aromatherapy, or even for midwives who are fully qualified aromatherapists, simply to monitor themselves, although self- and peer-evaluation can be valuable in its own right. Unfortunately, it is this lack of a sufficiently robust process of monitoring of midwifery aromatherapy at a corporate level which has led to various problems arising, as reported to this author in recent years. The eagerness of midwives to implement aromatherapy and other complementary therapies has created a power issue in which the individuals have sometimes lost sight of the reasons for incorporating complementary therapies into midwifery care (see Chapter 1).

The principles of supervision of midwives are to provide professional support, development and leadership in order to ensure protection of the public. Although the process of supervision may be removed from the statutory framework (Baird *et al.* 2015), the fundamental functions of the supervisory process are unlikely to change.

The aromatherapy monitoring process could be undertaken by a supervisor of midwives, or whatever role replaces it. The supervisor must have the relevant knowledge and experience, even when s/he is not actively involved in the implementation or provision of the aromatherapy service. There must be an opportunity for midwives to discuss any issues in an unbiased setting, but also to ensure that they reflect on, and learn from, their experiences of using aromatherapy and keep up to date through CPD (see above). Midwives could, for example, be required to complete one or two reflective case reports on their use of aromatherapy to discuss at their annual supervisory review. Where there is a group of midwives practising aromatherapy within a maternity unit, the supervisor could hold an annual or six-monthly group meeting to enable midwives to discuss cases in which aromatherapy has been successful and those in which it was less so, or where use of aromatherapy caused clinical or professional issues.

Escalating concerns

There must also be a framework within which midwives can bring to the notice of senior colleagues any concerns they have about the inappropriate use of aromatherapy in their unit. In its 2015 revision of *The Code*, the Nursing and Midwifery Council introduced a new clause requiring registrants to 'raise, and, if necessary, escalate any concerns about patient or public safety, or the level of care people are receiving' (NMC 2015, clause 16.1).

There are many situations involving the use of aromatherapy within midwifery practice which give great cause for concern. Midwives frequently seem not to recognise adequately that introducing aromatherapy into their care of women is an aspect of 'extended practice', which requires attention to all the relevant clauses in the NMC's various documents. This author often receives reports from midwives working in units which are failing to comply adequately with these requirements, and in some cases, are breaking the law. Examples include midwives blending oils for sale to women as a means of income generation, midwives blending batches of essential and carrier oils in their own homes for use by midwives in the unit, and others storing oil blends in a cupboard with open access, or even leaving the oils on a shelf accessible to all. There are also many maternity units which purport to have an 'aromatherapy service' in which there are no clinical guidelines (see later in the chapter). Further, despite midwives being required to be competent in all aspects of care, including complying with 'Essential Skills Cluster 5' in the *Standards for Pre-registration Midwifery Education* (NMC 2009) in order to mentor students adequately, many midwives do not fulfil these requirements.

Escalating concerns relating to the practice of aromatherapy by midwives is difficult since many senior managers and supervisors do not have any understanding of the pertinent issues. Added to this is the fact that aromatherapy, as with other complementary therapies, is not seen as a credible, viable or essential subject in either pre-registration or post-registration education, and is considered only as an option which some midwives may wish to explore once qualified. Where it is used, many professionals disregard the safety issues in the common belief that aromatherapy is simply aromatic massage. Further, there is no acknowledgement of the fact that women are using aromatherapy oils before and during pregnancy and birth, almost to epidemic proportions, and that this is causing increasing problems for midwives caring for women, especially in labour.

Indemnity insurance cover

The NMC *Code* clause 12 (NMC 2015) requires registrants to have in place an indemnity insurance arrangement which gives appropriate cover for any practice as a midwife in the United Kingdom. Midwives employed by the NHS who have been given permission to use aromatherapy in their practice will be covered by the maternity unit's vicarious liability insurance system.

A case was referred to the Nursing and Midwifery Council in 2009 in which a midwife, who was also an aromatherapist, but who had not been granted permission to use aromatherapy in her unit, gave an oil blend to a labouring mother who then mistakenly drank the liquid (BBC News 2009). Fortunately, the mother and baby suffered no adverse effects but the midwife was considered by the NMC Professional Conduct Committee to represent a continuing threat to women's safety and was removed from the register.

The Royal College of Midwives (RCM) currently provides medical malpractice insurance for full members employed by the NHS who offer private complementary therapy services 'on an occasional basis', on condition that they are appropriately qualified, competent and working within the parameters of NMC regulations. The definition of 'occasional' is not clear, but it is presumed that any midwife working fewer hours in private practice than in NHS employment would be covered, although this should be checked on an individual basis.

Midwives working for private institutions which have a link to the NHS will also be covered directly by the RCM insurance policy, although those employed by general practitioners will not as these services are outside the NHS contracting system. Those employed by a private company or institution will generally be covered by the company's own indemnity insurance policy. The RCM does not cover midwives working in full-time self-employment providing private maternity aromatherapy, and these midwives must make alternative insurance arrangements. This will necessitate accessing training which is both maternity specific and accredited by an organisation linked to an appropriate insurance company.

Similarly, the Royal College of Nursing (RCN) provides cover for anyone working within the NHS but seems rather more flexible on the subject of complementary therapies in private practice, on condition that midwives are full members of the RCN. Full membership of the RCM with associate membership of the RCN does not provide suitable insurance cover. The RCN covers individuals who have established their own business, in terms of the clinical health and social care services they provide, but this insurance is invalidated if the member takes on another health professional in the practice – in this case, corporate insurance cover would be required.

Midwives are covered by the RCN for private antenatal and postnatal services but this does not extend to care during labour, nor are other practices, notably those involving incisions such as frenulotomy or circumcision, included. Fetal ultrasound scanning and lactation consultancy are also excluded. Antenatal classes are covered on condition that there is an individual care plan for each person attending the class. Where midwives are running private or NHS antenatal classes on the use of massage and aromatherapy, they must take care with logistical issues such as health and safety, and must not use essential oils in the classes, nor should they allow women to 'sniff' the aromas, or provide ready-blended aromatherapy oils for women to purchase/be given for home use.

In respect of evidence-based complementary therapies, the RCN covers the use of aromatherapy essential oils when used within recognised health or social care settings, as well as acupuncture, hypnotherapy and massage, but does not cover homeopathy under any circumstances. Members must have a recognised qualification in the therapy and work within the NMC parameters for safe professional practice. In reality, midwives with a full qualification in a particular complementary therapy, such as homeopathy, will be able to obtain indemnity insurance cover from their therapy's professional organisation. However, some midwifery aromatherapy courses are accredited by other organisations such as the Federation of Antenatal Educators, so that midwives and doulas who have completed specifically identified training courses can obtain insurance cover for private maternity-specific aromatherapy practice, even though they are not fully qualified aromatherapists.

Clinical guidelines

In the NHS and in many private organisations it is mandatory to have local clinical guidelines to set out precisely what the maternity aromatherapy service will involve. This is not only to protect the mothers and babies but also the midwives practising aromatherapy. It may be appropriate to specify named midwives who are permitted to use aromatherapy – perhaps with a two-tier system of those who are fully trained to use essential oils autonomously and those who have received a shorter in-house training to use a limited selection of oils or just pre-blended oils. It may also be wise to maintain a list of the approved midwives, with criteria for due dates of CPD, and situations in which their 'live' status on the register is maintained or discontinued. For example, midwives may circulate around the maternity unit to areas where they are not able to use aromatherapy, so should be required to undertake some updating prior to resuming their aromatherapy practice on returning to those clinical areas where essential oils are in use.

If essential oils are to be used by midwives both in the unit and in the community, there may need to be differentiated criteria to cover issues such as storage and transport of oils by community midwives. The specific essential oils which are permitted for use should be identified and there should ideally be a profile summary of each oil, perhaps as an appendix to the guideline, which outlines the chemical constituents, indications, contraindications and precautions and the other oils with which each oil can be blended. It may be necessary to specify a gestation before which essential oils cannot be used – for example, if an intrapartum service is planned, this may relate only to term labours from 37 weeks gestation. Where relatively low- to moderately high-risk women may be labouring in the main delivery suite but are able to receive aromatherapy, the guideline may need to specify issues such as avoiding certain high-risk rooms or discontinuing aromatherapy once syntocinon is commenced.

It may also be worth considering including a point related to midwives' responsibilities when women bring in their own oils for use in labour, or when they wish to be accompanied by an independent therapist or birth supporter who uses essential oils. In these cases, issues such as expected lines of communication and checking indemnity insurance and Disclosure and Barring Service (DBS) clearance may need to be identified. It is the mother's prerogative to invite a practitioner to accompany her, but the therapist must understand her obligations to the mother and the maternity unit. Mothers labouring in their own homes are, of course, entitled to have with them whomever they choose, but the therapist will still need to acknowledge the legal requirements that the midwife retains overall responsibility for the mother's care.

It is also essential to cross-reference the aromatherapy guidelines to other clinical guidelines – for example, those for pain relief in labour, epidural anaesthesia, induction of labour and preterm labour. Midwives should also refer to other documents on issues such as administration of medicines, infection control, health and safety and manual handling.

Suggestions for the points to be covered in a unit guideline on the use of aromatherapy in midwifery practice are given in Box 5.5. These suggestions relate only to the specific issues related to aromatherapy, and midwives will, of course, take steps to ensure that any local requisites are also included.

Box 5.5 Points to include in aromatherapy clinical guidelines

Policy statement (mission statement)

Definition of aromatherapy and massage

Rationale for implementing/using aromatherapy and massage in midwifery practice – for example, reducing intervention, aiding normality, pain relief – this may need to be balanced against national recommendations such as the NICE intrapartum guideline (NICE 2014b) (see Chapter 1)

Benefits of aromatherapy and massage in pregnancy, labour, puerperium, as appropriate to the intended service, evidence-based with contemporary research references (see Chapter 2)

Approved training accepted as suitable for midwives intending to use aromatherapy in their practice, including external (national/international) and in-house requirements

CPD requirements related to maternity
aromatherapy – suitable activities, frequency

Requirements for newly employed midwives
joining the unit (induction session)

Requirement for aromatherapy practice by midwives
to be based upon sound principles, available knowledge
and skill and, where possible, based on contemporary
evidence and/or authoritative debate (see Chapter 3)

Requirement for midwives to be able to justify decisions
regarding the administration of aromatherapy and massage

Maintenance of a 'live' register of midwives approved
to administer essential oils and massage and criteria for
remaining on the register (e.g. time since last use)

Supervision/mentoring of midwifery practice in
relation to aromatherapy and massage

Mothers who are eligible to receive aromatherapy and massage

Indications for aromatherapy and massage
in pregnancy, labour, puerperium

Contraindications and precautions (see Chapter 4)

Administration – percentage blends permitted; assessment of individual

Specific issues related to individual oils (e.g. clary sage not to
be used with syntocinon; no use of oils in birthing pool, etc.)

Methods of administration; specific contraindications (e.g. use of
vaporisers/diffusers; essential oils not to be used in antenatal classes)

Essential oils suggested for specific conditions (see Chapter 6)

Consent, confidentiality, record-keeping

Audit and evaluation

Health and safety issues

Profiles of essential oils to be used in the service,
evidence-based (see Chapter 7)

Protocols for specific oil blends, if appropriate

Evaluating the maternity aromatherapy service

It is important to evaluate the success, effectiveness and cost-effectiveness of the aromatherapy service from the outset. This can be done by collating referrals on the computerised notes system or by devising a form which accompanies aromatherapy treatment notes, to be completed and forwarded to the midwife responsible for managing the service. Statistics should be collected to be analysed at the end of a specified period, and may include the number of women using the aromatherapy service, indications for use, and other information relating to its use. For example, if aromatherapy is offered in the birth centre, details of the labours of women using essential oils should be recorded, such as length of labour, use of other analgesia and oxytocics, birth outcome (normal delivery/forceps/Caesarean, etc.), Apgar score in the baby, transfer to main delivery suite/neonatal unit. An evaluation questionnaire could also be given to mothers who have used aromatherapy, to determine their satisfaction with the service, with another for the staff involved in administering the aromatherapy treatments. Production of an annual report to be sent to midwifery managers, obstetricians or other senior staff as appropriate may demonstrate the success of the service and justify its continuation, particularly if cost issues are raised.

Chapter 6

Application of Aromatherapy to Maternity Care

This chapter provides a ready reference for clinical practice. The chart on pages 147–159 gives suggestions for essential oils which are suitable for the treatment of specific conditions (column 1). Suitable essential oils which may have a direct therapeutic effect (column 2) are supported by suggestions of other essential oils which could be used in an aromatic blend to treat a woman with the condition (column 3). The percentage dose (column 4) relates to doses for massage. A guide to suitable methods of administration, relevant to the condition, is given (column 5), together with safety information and general comments (column 6). The carrier oil has not been specified, but grapeseed or sweet almond oil are the most versatile (check women are not allergic to almonds). Several case studies from clinical practice are given at the end of the chapter to illustrate suggested treatment regimens.

Midwives, doulas and other caregivers should adhere to the principles for safe practice, namely:

- Dosages should be kept to a maximum of 1.5% in pregnancy, 2% in labour and postnatally, with 3% being permissible for 'natural induction' for post-dates pregnancy (see Chapter 2).

- A maximum of three essential oils should be used in any one blend (see Chapter 2).

- Women should be assessed for safety aspects prior to treatment – if an essential oil is contraindicated, select an alternative (see Chapter 4).

- If in any doubt, the use of essential oils should be restricted, but the mother may be able to have a massage with carrier oil only.

- Comprehensive records should be maintained of all treatments given (see Chapter 5).

Table 6.1 Aromatherapy treatment for pregnancy, labour and postnatal conditions

CONDITION	ESSENTIAL OILS – DIRECT	ESSENTIAL OILS – BLENDING	DOSE FOR MASSAGE	SUGGESTED METHOD	COMMENTS
Appetite changes	Bergamot, black pepper, grapefruit, lime, peppermint, spearmint	Cypress, eucalyptus, frankincense, mandarin/tangerine, neroli, orange	0.5–1%	Neck and shoulder massage Hand or foot massage In the bath	Indirect treatment only – do not use by mouth 4–6 drops in 2 ml carrier oil for the bath Beware link between taste and olfactory system – sense of smell changes as pregnancy progresses
Backache	Black pepper, lavender for pain relief Chamomile, frankincense, geranium, ylang ylang to relax	Bergamot, eucalyptus, grapefruit, lime, mandarin/tangerine, neroli, orange, peppermint, rose, spearmint	1.5% in pregnancy 2% in labour and postnatally	Back massage, with mother upright or on side In the bath As a compress over affected area	Use minimal black pepper – strong aroma Care needed with sacral massage in early pregnancy Apply firm sacral pressure in labour 4–6 drops in 2 ml carrier oil 2–3 drops in a litre of warm/cold water for compress Avoid rose until 34 weeks gestation *See Case study 6.1*

CONDITION	ESSENTIAL OILS – DIRECT	ESSENTIAL OILS – BLENDING	DOSE FOR MASSAGE	SUGGESTED METHOD	COMMENTS
Breast discomfort (postnatal)	Cypress for engorgement Geranium to aid lactation Black pepper for pain relief	Chamomile, eucalyptus, frankincense, jasmine, lavender, rose, ylang ylang	1.5% in pregnancy 2% postnatally	Back or foot massage	4–6 drops in 2 ml carrier for the bath
				In the bath	Wash breasts with clear water before baby feeds
	Bergamot, grapefruit, lime, mandarin/ tangerine, neroli, orange for relaxation			Compress direct to breasts for engorgement	2–3 drops in a litre of warm/ cold water for compress Do not generally apply directly to breasts – if compress is used, mother should wash breasts with clean water to avoid ingestion by baby when feeding
Caesarean section recovery	Black pepper, lavender for pain relief Frankincense, rose, ylang ylang for relaxation Peppermint, spearmint for intestinal transit Lavender, tea tree for wound healing	Bergamot, eucalyptus, geranium, grapefruit, jasmine, lime, mandarin/tangerine, neroli, orange	2%	Foot, hand or back massage for pain relief and relaxation	Massage depends on mother's tolerance and mobility
				Clockwise massage to arches of feet for constipation and paralytic ileus	Arches of feet correspond to reflexology zones for intestines
				In the bath for wound healing	4–6 drops in 2 ml carrier oil for the bath Bath water must cover wound area – dry carefully afterwards

Condition	Essential oils	Dilution	Methods	Notes
Carpal tunnel syndrome	Cypress, lime, geranium for fluid retention Black pepper, lavender for pain relief Peppermint to stimulate circulation	Chamomile, eucalyptus, frankincense, mandarin/tangerine, neroli, orange, rose, spearmint, ylang ylang	1% in pregnancy 2% postnatally	Hand and arm massage Compress around entire area	Massage from fingers towards heart, plus shoulder and neck massage 2–3 drops in a litre of warm/cold water for compress Avoid rose until 34 weeks gestation *See Case study 6.3*
Constipation	Bergamot, grapefruit, lime, mandarin/tangerine, neroli, orange to aid gastrointestinal tract motility Black pepper to stimulate intestines	Chamomile, eucalyptus, frankincense, geranium, jasmine, lavender, peppermint, rose, spearmint, ylang ylang	1–1.5% in pregnancy 2% postnatally	Clockwise massage of arches of feet Back massage Abdominal compress In the bath	Arches of feet correspond to reflexology zones for intestines Avoid jasmine in pregnancy, avoid rose until 34 weeks gestation 4–6 drops in 2 ml carrier oil for compress 4–6 drops in 2 ml carrier oil for bath *See Case study 6.2*
Coughs, colds, sinus congestion	Cypress, eucalyptus, frankincense, lavender as decongestant Clary sage can be used in postnatal period if lochia normal Tea tree as anti-infective	Bergamot, black pepper, chamomile, geranium, grapefruit, lime, mandarin/tangerine, neroli, orange, peppermint, rose, spearmint, ylang ylang	0.5–1% in pregnancy 2% postnatally	Inhalation with steam for coughs, colds Gentle facial massage of sinus areas with 0.5% blend Facial spray in water Aromastick™	Take care with hot water (health and safety) Low dose to avoid excessively strong aroma close to nostrils 2 drops in 500 ml cold water for facial spray – keep in fridge Discard water-based blend after 24 hours Aromastick™ to be used with caution – 2 drops essential oil only

CONDITION	ESSENTIAL OILS – DIRECT	ESSENTIAL OILS – BLENDING	DOSE FOR MASSAGE	SUGGESTED METHOD	COMMENTS
Cramp, restless legs	Black pepper, lavender, neroli for pain relief Cypress, geranium for oedema Peppermint, spearmint to freshen and stimulate feet and legs	Bergamot, chamomile, eucalyptus, frankincense, grapefruit, lime, mandarin/tangerine, neroli, orange, ylang ylang	1–1.5% in pregnancy 2% postnatally	Compress around legs Leg and foot massage In the bath	2–3 drops in a litre of warm/cold water for compress, using large towel or tea towel Massage from toes towards groin 4–6 drops in 2 ml carrier oil for bath Bath water should cover legs
Cystitis	Chamomile, eucalyptus, tea tree for anti-infective effects Cypress for effects on fluid balance Black pepper, lavender for discomfort and pain	Bergamot, clary sage, eucalyptus, frankincense, geranium, grapefruit, jasmine, lime, mandarin/tangerine, neroli, orange, peppermint, rose, spearmint, tea tree, ylang ylang	1–1.5% in pregnancy 2% postnatally	Back massage In the bath In the bidet Vulval wash Suprapubic compress	4–6 drops in 2 ml carrier oil for bath 2–4 drops in bidet water after micturition 2–4 drops in a litre cold/warm water, sluiced down from pubis whilst sitting over toilet or bidet as vulval wash 2–3 drops in a litre warm/cold water for compress Ensure not a severe urinary tract infection requiring antibiotics

Depression	Clary sage, jasmine for postnatal depression Frankincense to calm Bergamot, grapefruit, mandarin/tangerine, neroli, orange to uplift Lavender to relax	Black pepper, eucalyptus, peppermint, rose, spearmint	1% in pregnancy 2% postnatally	Full body massage, or hand, foot or back massage In the bath	Massage should be brisk and light, not deep and slow, to avoid exacerbating depression 4–6 drops in 2 ml carrier oil for bath Do not use ylang ylang – may cause mother to become too introspective Avoid clary sage, jasmine in pregnancy
Diarrhoea	Black pepper, chamomile, neroli, peppermint, spearmint to reduce colonic spasm Tea tree if infective	Bergamot, cypress, eucalyptus, frankincense, geranium, grapefruit, jasmine, lavender, lime, mandarin/ tangerine, orange, rose	1–1.5% in pregnancy 2% postnatally	Abdominal and sacral compress In the bath Back massage	2–3 drops in a litre of warm/ cold water for compress 4–6 drops in 2 ml carrier oil for bath Seek medical advice if infective
Epidural recovery	Black pepper, lavender for general pain relief Lavender, peppermint for headache Chamomile, ylang ylang for muscle relaxation	Bergamot, eucalyptus, frankincense, geranium, grapefruit, lime, mandarin/ tangerine, neroli, orange, peppermint, rose, spearmint	2%	Neck, shoulders and upper back massage In the bath Foot bath Shoulder compress	Avoid massage to lower back until cannula entry point has healed, or cover wound 4–6 drops in 2 ml carrier oil for bath 2–3 drops in bowl of water for foot bath 2–3 drops in a litre of warm/ cold water for compress

CONDITION	ESSENTIAL OILS – DIRECT	ESSENTIAL OILS – BLENDING	DOSE FOR MASSAGE	SUGGESTED METHOD	COMMENTS
Haemorrhoids	Cypress, geranium, lime for astringent properties Lavender to relieve discomfort and promote relaxation Tea tree for prevention of infection	Bergamot, black pepper, chamomile, eucalyptus, frankincense, grapefruit, mandarin/tangerine, neroli, orange, peppermint, rose, spearmint, ylang ylang	1–1.5% in pregnancy 2% postnatally	Bidet In the bath Spray for direct application	2–3 drops in bidet water 4–6 drops in 2 ml carrier oil for bath 2 drops in 250 ml water for spray Discard water-based blend after 24 hours Avoid rose until 34 weeks gestation *See Case study 6.2*
Headache	Black pepper, lavender, peppermint for pain relief Bergamot, chamomile, ylang ylang for deep relaxation Peppermint, spearmint, lime, grapefruit for nausea	Cypress, eucalyptus, frankincense, geranium, jasmine, mandarin/tangerine, neroli, orange, rose	0.5–1% in pregnancy 2% in labour or postnatally	Compress over affected area Neck, shoulders and upper back massage Head massage without oils	2–3 drops in a litre of warm/cold water for compress Woman with migraine should not generally receive essential oils – massage can be done with carrier oil only Be alert to risk of severe pre-eclampsia
Heartburn and indigestion	Bergamot, black pepper, chamomile, peppermint, spearmint	Eucalyptus, frankincense, geranium, grapefruit, lavender, lime, mandarin/tangerine, neroli, orange, rose	1–1.5% in pregnancy 2% postnatally	Foot, hand, back massage Gentle abdominal massage	Avoid abdominal massage if anteriorly situated placenta Avoid rose until 34 weeks gestation

Hypertension	Chamomile, clary sage, lavender, ylang ylang – hypotensive effect Frankincense, geranium to calm and relax	Bergamot, black pepper, geranium, grapefruit, jasmine, lime, mandarin/ tangerine, neroli, orange, peppermint, rose, spearmint	1% in pregnancy 2% postnatally	Massage – back, foot, hand, full body In the bath Foot bath	Avoid clary sage in pregnancy Avoid rose until 34 weeks gestation Be alert to severe pre-eclampsia 4–6 drops in 2 ml carrier oil for bath 2–3 drops in bowl of water for foot bath
Induction/ acceleration of labour	Clary sage, jasmine, lavender to promote labour, frankincense, neroli, ylang ylang to relax	Bergamot, black pepper, chamomile, cypress, eucalyptus, geranium, grapefruit, lime, mandarin/ tangerine, orange, peppermint, rose, spearmint	3% for natural induction only 2% for acceleration in established labour	Massage – back, foot, hand In the bath	Avoid clary sage until cause of delay/prolonged labour is known 4–6 drops in 2 ml carrier oil for bath Practitioner must, under EU law, undertake the first treatment – remainder of blend can be given for use at home for induction if properly labelled (see Chapter 5) Avoid tea tree – may relax uterus
Insomnia, tiredness, fatigue	Chamomile, lavender, ylang ylang – sedative Frankincense – calming Jasmine if with postnatal depression/blues Eucalyptus, peppermint, spearmint to uplift and stimulate during the day	Bergamot, black pepper, cypress, geranium, grapefruit, lavender, lime, mandarin/tangerine, neroli, orange, rose	1–1.5% in pregnancy 2% postnatally	Massage – back, foot, hand, full body In the bath 1 drop of essential oil on a tissue left on pillow	Best given in the evening 4–6 drops in 2 ml carrier oil for bath Avoid direct application of oils to pillow – oxidisation will occur before the following night Avoid rose until 34 weeks gestation

CONDITION	ESSENTIAL OILS – DIRECT	ESSENTIAL OILS – BLENDING	DOSE FOR MASSAGE	SUGGESTED METHOD	COMMENTS
Lactation, insufficient	Geranium, sweet fennel for let-down reflex Geranium, cypress for engorgement Frankincense, jasmine, ylang ylang to calm	Bergamot, eucalyptus, grapefruit, lavender, lime, mandarin/ tangerine, neroli, orange, peppermint, rose, spearmint	2%	In the bath Foot, hand, back massage	4–6 drops in 2 ml carrier oil for bath Do not have baby in bathroom Do not massage breasts unless engorgement present NB Sweet fennel should not be used in pregnancy and has limited uses in labour and the postnatal period. It is therefore not profiled in this book but could be added to the practitioner's selection of essential oils on completion of an evidence-based profile for breastfeeding issues
Latent phase of labour	Clary sage, jasmine, lavender to promote contractions Frankincense to calm Chamomile to aid rest Black pepper, lavender for pain relief	Bergamot, cypress, eucalyptus, geranium, grapefruit, lime, mandarin/ tangerine, neroli, orange, peppermint, rose, spearmint, ylang ylang	2%	Massage – back, foot, hand In the bath Suprapubic compress	Avoid tea tree in labour, may relax uterus 4–6 drops in 2 ml carrier oil for bath 2–3 drops in 500 ml warm/ cold water for compress NB NICE (2014b) intrapartum guidelines do not recommend aromatherapy for latent phase of labour – be prepared to defend decision

Condition	Recommended oils	Oils to avoid	Dilution	Application	Cautions/notes
Libido, reduced	Ylang ylang, rose as aphrodisiac Frankincense to calm Lavender, chamomile to aid relaxation Geranium to balance Citrus oils to lift mood	Black pepper, cypress, eucalyptus, jasmine, peppermint, spearmint	1–1.5% in pregnancy 2% postnatally	Massage – foot, hand, back, full body In the bath	Avoid jasmine in pregnancy Avoid rose until 34 weeks gestation 4–6 drops in 2 ml carrier oil for bath
Ligament, groin pain	Black pepper, lavender for pain relief Chamomile, frankincense, ylang ylang for muscle relaxation	Bergamot, cypress, eucalyptus, geranium, grapefruit, lime, mandarin/tangerine, neroli, orange, peppermint, rose, spearmint	1–1.5% in pregnancy 2% postnatally	Massage – foot and leg, back In the bath	Avoid rose until 34 weeks gestation 4–6 drops in 2 ml carrier oil for bath Water should cover groin area
Nausea and vomiting	Bergamot, grapefruit, lime, peppermint, spearmint for anti-emetic effect	Black pepper, frankincense, geranium, mandarin/tangerine, neroli, orange, ylang ylang	0.5–1% in pregnancy 2% in labour or postnatally	Massage – back, foot, hand In the bath On tissue, cotton wool ball, gauze swab – 2 drops neat oil	Many women will not want aromatherapy with pregnancy sickness as they may be very sensitive to odours – if the woman agrees to aromatherapy treatment, it is wise to use just 1–2 essential oils and possibly only 0.5% 4–6 drops in 2 ml carrier oil for bath Not suitable for the chronic nausea of pregnancy Good for labour and postnatal in-patient stay – inhale when surges of nausea occur

CONDITION	ESSENTIAL OILS – DIRECT	ESSENTIAL OILS – BLENDING	DOSE FOR MASSAGE	SUGGESTED METHOD	COMMENTS
Neck and shoulder pain	Black pepper, lavender for pain relief Chamomile, ylang ylang for muscular relaxation Frankincense to aid coping strategies	Bergamot, cypress, eucalyptus, geranium, grapefruit, lime, mandarin/tangerine, neroli, orange, peppermint, rose, spearmint	1–1.5% in pregnancy 2% postnatally	Neck, shoulder, upper back massage Head massage without oils Compress around shoulders In the bath	2–3 drops in 500 ml warm/cold water for compress 4–6 drops in 2 ml carrier oil for bath
Oedema of legs and feet	Cypress, bergamot, lime, geranium for fluid retention Black pepper, lavender for pain relief	Chamomile, eucalyptus, frankincense, grapefruit, mandarin/tangerine, neroli, orange, peppermint, rose, spearmint, tea tree, ylang ylang	1–1.5% in pregnancy 2% postnatally	Compress around legs In the bath Massage – legs and feet	2–3 drops in 500 ml warm/cold water for compress 4–6 drops in 2 ml carrier oil for bath Rest with legs raised afterwards Massage from feet to groin if possible, taking care if skin very over-stretched – compress may be more comfortable Avoid rose until 34 weeks gestation *See Case study 6.3*

Pain relief in labour	Black pepper, clary sage, jasmine, lavender for direct pain relief Frankincense to calm Any citrus oils to lift mood and aid coping strategies	Bergamot, chamomile, cypress, eucalyptus, geranium, grapefruit, lime, mandarin/tangerine, neroli, orange, peppermint, rose, spearmint, ylang ylang	2%	Massage – lower back, foot In the bath Abdominal or suprapubic compress	**Avoid clary sage if contractions well-established** 4–6 drops in 2 ml carrier oil for bath Do not add essential oils directly to bath water if membranes ruptured Do not add essential oils directly to birthing pool 2–3 drops in 500 ml warm/cold water for compress NB NICE (2014b) intrapartum guidelines do not recommend aromatherapy for pain relief in labour – be prepared to defend decision See Case study 6.4
Pelvic girdle/ symphysis pubis pain	Black pepper, lavender for pain relief Chamomile, lavender, ylang ylang for muscle relaxation Frankincense, ylang ylang to calm and relax	Bergamot, cypress, eucalyptus, geranium, grapefruit, lime, mandarin/tangerine, neroli, orange, peppermint, rose, spearmint	1–1.5% in pregnancy 2% postnatally	Back and leg massage Suprapubic compress In the bath if able to get in Foot bath (indirect)	2–3 drops in 500 ml warm/cold water for compress 4–6 drops in 2 ml carrier oil for bath Bath water should cover up to waist 2–3 drops in water for foot bath See Case study 6.1

CONDITION	ESSENTIAL OILS – DIRECT	ESSENTIAL OILS – BLENDING	DOSE FOR MASSAGE	SUGGESTED METHOD	COMMENTS
Perineal wound healing	Cypress, lavender, tea tree for wound healing Lavender, black pepper for pain relief	Use only essential oils appropriate for wound healing, others may cause sensitivity	2%	In the bath Bidet Vulval wash	4–6 drops in 2 ml carrier oil for bath 2–3 drops in bidet water Wound must be thoroughly dried after water-based treatment Check woman does not become sensitive to tea tree Do not apply any oils direct to perineum nor to a sanitary pad – wound care must be based on contemporary research evidence
Retained placenta	Clary sage for direct effect	Jasmine, lavender	2%	Compress – to abdomen or suprapubic area Inhalation	2–3 drops in 250 ml warm/cold water for compress 1–2 drops neat on tissue for inhalation Only to be used with caution in third stage of labour NOT to be used for retained products Ensure all normal midwifery care attended to first Be alert to blood loss

Condition	Recommendations	Essential oils	Dilution	Method	Dosage
Skin itching	Chamomile, peppermint, spearmint	Black pepper, geranium, lavender	1%	In the bath Compress	3–4 drops in 2 ml carrier oil for bath 2–3 drops in 500 ml warm/cold water for compress if localised to small area Differential diagnosis – check for cholestasis gravidarum
Stress, anxiety, fear, tension	Frankincense to calm Ylang ylang, lavender, geranium, to relax Chamomile to aid rest Citrus oils to uplift mood	Black pepper, cypress, eucalyptus, peppermint, rose, spearmint	1.5% in pregnancy 2% postnatally	Massage – foot, hand, back, whole body Inhalation of frankincense for acute stress (e.g. having blood taken, hearing bad news)	Repeated treatments provide an accumulative effect in chronic stress 2 drops on tissue for inhalation
Vaginal discharge	Bergamot, lavender, tea tree to prevent/aid treatment of infection Tea tree or any citrus oils as deodorizer if necessary	Use only essential oils appropriate as anti-infective agents – others may cause sensitivity	1%	In the bath In the bidet Vulval wash	4–6 drops in 2 ml carrier oil for bath 2–3 drops in bidet water 2–3 drops in 500 ml warm/cold water, to sluice area whilst sitting on toilet or bidet
Varicose veins	Cypress, geranium for astringent properties Peppermint, spearmint, eucalyptus to refresh legs Black pepper, lavender for pain relief	Bergamot, chamomile, frankincense, grapefruit, lime, mandarin/tangerine, neroli, orange, rose, tea tree, ylang ylang	1.5% in pregnancy 2% postnatally	Compress In the bath In the bidet	2–3 drops in warm/cold water for compress 2–3 drops in 2 ml carrier oil for bath 4–6 drops in bidet water Water should cover affected area Bidet and bath both suitable for vulval varicosities

Case study 6.1 Backache and symphysis pubis discomfort

Clara was 37 years old and 33 weeks pregnant with her first child. She was generally fit and well and before her pregnancy, she normally went to the gym four times a week because she had a very sedentary job as a secretary in London. Clara was feeling very tired, and her commute to and from work exacerbated this because she was often unable to find a seat and had to stand for the 50-minute journey. She was rarely visiting the gym now, especially as she had developed nagging lumbosacral backache and pain in the suprapubic region.

When Clara visited the midwifery complementary therapies clinic, she was exhausted and miserable. The midwife's compassion caused Clara to burst into tears – at last someone seemed to understand how she was feeling. After taking a history, the midwife felt that Clara needed to be treated holistically so that both her physical discomforts and her emotional state could be improved. She asked Clara if she would be able to take some time off work, or work from home for a few days in order to avoid the difficult commute. The midwife also asked her to check her seating at work and, if possible, to request an ergonomic chair which could support her back more effectively. She arranged an appointment with the physiotherapist for some suggested easy exercises which might ease the backache and pelvic pain, and also gave Clara advice about sitting, lifting, lying in bed and avoiding abducting her legs in order to relieve the pelvic pain.

The midwife felt that Clara could benefit from an aromatherapy massage and Clara was enthusiastic about this. After consideration of the appropriate essential oils, the midwife suggested a blend of black pepper for pain relief, lavender for additional pain relief and also relaxation, plus ylang ylang for physical and emotional relaxation. When offered the three essential oils to smell, Clara did not like the black pepper, which she felt was too strong and preferred the midwife's suggested alternative of peppermint to refresh and uplift her. The midwife blended 25 ml grapeseed oil with 2 drops of lavender, 2 drops of ylang ylang and 1 drop of peppermint, giving a 1% blend appropriate for pregnancy.

With Clara seated on a stool and leaning on pillows piled high on the clinic couch, the midwife was able to perform a back massage for about 20 minutes. She gave attention to Clara's neck and shoulders and to her lower back, although she was careful not to apply too much firm localised thumb pressure to the area over the sacral foramen as she knew that this could potentially trigger labour. Clara enjoyed the massage and felt much better at the end. She was delighted to be offered another appointment for the following week.

The midwife also suggested that she could give Clara the remainder of the oil blend to take home for use in the bath, but Clara said she was unable to get into the bath. The midwife therefore gave Clara instructions on how her partner could give her a short massage, or how she could make a warm compress with some of the blend to apply to the lumbosacral area. Clara was given written information about how to use the oil blend and after-care advice about drinking plenty of water, 'listening to her body' and relaxing when necessary, as well as a telephone number to call the midwife in the event of any concerns.

NB This client's treatment also included some reflex zone therapy of the feet, prior to the aromatherapy back massage (see Tiran 2010b).

Case study 6.2 Constipation and haemorrhoids

Michelle was 34 weeks pregnant and expecting her second baby. She had been referred to the midwives' complementary therapy clinic with severe constipation. She had always been prone to constipation, her normal bowel activity being every second or third day, but it had worsened considerably in pregnancy and especially in the last few weeks. On the advice of her named midwife, she had tried dietary changes, increasing her fluid intake and taking gentle laxatives, but to no avail. She was now only having a bowel movement about once a week and was very uncomfortable.

The midwife suggested that a foot massage might be helpful, using aromatherapy oils but focusing on the arches of the feet which, in reflexology principles, relate to the intestines. They agreed on a 1% blend of geranium, grapefruit and cypress, prepared in 25 ml carrier oil, with three drops of grapefruit and one each of the geranium and cypress. The midwife gave Michelle an all-over foot massage but concentrated on clockwise massage on the arches of the feet, using very firm thumb pressure and then her knuckles, with her hand in a fist.

Following the treatment, Michelle was given the remainder of the blend with written instructions on how her partner could treat her with a daily foot massage, together with the normal after-care advice. Michelle was also advised to use the blend in the bath daily – the midwife explained that the oils need to be in contact with the haemorrhoids in order for their astringent (tightening) action to take effect.

The midwife telephoned Michelle three days later and was pleased to hear that Michelle felt a little less uncomfortable and had had two bowel movements since the massage. She was continuing to use a small amount in the bath for her haemorrhoids, and her partner massaged her feet each evening. Her haemorrhoids were certainly less irritating and she had found that having a quick bath with the oils immediately after having a bowel movement seemed to reduce the pain.

Case study 6.3 Oedema of legs and carpal tunnel syndrome

Thandi, a 28-year-old primigravida, was 36 weeks pregnant. She had commenced pregnancy with a body mass index of 30 and, despite careful monitoring and supervision of her diet and exercise, her appetite was voracious and she had gained considerably more weight, particularly in the third trimester. Her feet and legs, as far as her calves, were now very oedematous, although her blood pressure remained stable with a diastolic of around 85. When Thandi was seen by the midwife, she was also complaining of pain and tingling in her left wrist and hand and was unable to perform fine motor tasks with that hand.

The midwife suggested an aromatherapy treatment to help both the leg oedema and the carpal tunnel syndrome. Following discussion with Thandi, a 1.5% blend of 3 drops of cypress, 4 drops of lime and 2 drops of peppermint oil was prepared in 30 ml of grapeseed carrier oil. The midwife started by applying a compress of the blend to Thandi's left hand, which was left in place for the duration of the treatment. She then performed a foot and leg massage, using upwards stroking movements with both hands, in an attempt to encourage return of the excess fluid to the lymphatic system. Initially it was quite uncomfortable for Thandi because the skin on her legs was very tight, so the midwife used light pressure; then, once Thandi reported that it was no longer painful, she increased the pressure, using a very firm movement. The massage was performed for about seven minutes on each leg and foot, and both Thandi and the midwife were pleased to observe a reasonable reduction in swelling at the end. On removing the compress from Thandi's left hand, the difference in swelling was astounding. Thandi could now move her fingers and the pain had reduced to a manageable level.

As only about 8 ml of the oil blend had been used for the massage, the midwife was able to give the remainder of the blend to Thandi to take home. Thandi was given written instructions on how to apply a compress to both her arm and her legs and then to rest with her feet raised for at least 20 minutes, once a day.

Case study 6.4 Care in labour

Annabel was a primigravida at 39 weeks and 4 days gestation. She had arrived at the birthing centre, having been contracting irregularly every 5–8 minutes for the last three hours. She was very anxious but coping reasonably well with the contractions. Her midwife met her and admitted her to a birthing room to take the history and complete the necessary observations. No examination *per vaginam* was performed but it was concluded that Annabel was not yet in fully established labour. However she did not want to go home.

The midwife suggested that, since the membranes were intact, Annabel might like to have a bath with essential oils, to relax her. Following discussion, Annabel chose rose and lavender for relaxation, pain relief and to aid progress, and frankincense to calm her. This was prepared as a 2% blend in 10 ml carrier oil, using 1 drop each of the lavender and frankincense and 2 drops of rose; about 5 ml was added to the bath water. Annabel relaxed in the bath for about 35 minutes, with the warm water being topped up halfway through, and then chose to get out. She seemed much calmer and the contractions were becoming much more regular – about every three minutes. She was advised to remain active for as long as possible, and enjoyed using the birthing ball and the rope.

After another hour or so, Annabel was feeling the contractions much more intensely and asked for some pain relief although she wanted to continue to lean over the birthing ball. The midwife suggested that Annabel could have a back massage, and she liked this idea. The contractions were now well established, so the midwife excluded clary sage and jasmine oils, and instead offered black pepper for pain relief and bergamot and neroli to relax and uplift Annabel, who agreed that these smelled very pleasant. The midwife prepared a 2% blend, using 1 drop of black pepper, 1 drop of neroli and 2 drops of bergamot in 10 ml of carrier oil. As Annabel was becoming rather anxious and agitated again, the midwife also gave her 1 drop of neat frankincense, massaged lightly into the centre of the palms of her two hands. (Frankincense is 'the ultimate calmer' and the centre of the palm is a reflexology relaxation point.) The midwife then performed a back massage for about ten minutes, focusing particularly on the lower back and using firm thumb pressure in the area over the sacral foramen for pain relief. Annabel asked the midwife to stop massaging during contractions but was happy for her to apply very firm pressure to the sacrum at this time.

Annabel wanted to continue with the back massage, especially the sacral pressure during contractions, and the midwife showed her partner, Jim, how to do this so that she could complete her observations and records. Jim was particularly sensitive and felt he was doing something useful by helping with the massage. Labour progressed well, and Annabel entered the transition stage just an hour and a half later. At this point she became agitated again and starting asking for an epidural, but the midwife's calm reassurance and Jim's continuing love and attention persuaded her that this was not necessary. As Annabel had decided to sit on the bed, the midwife suggested some gentle, very light effleurage (stroking) massage of her abdomen, using a different blend which could be more effective. A 2% blend of 1 drop of black pepper and 1 drop of lavender in 5 ml of grapeseed carrier oil was prepared and the midwife used this to massage Annabel's abdomen, thighs and hips. She also gave her another single drop of neat frankincense massaged into the centre of her hands to keep her calm.

All of a sudden, Annabel wanted to lean over the birthing ball again and said that she was ready to push. Fifteen minutes later, Annabel gave birth to a beautiful baby girl, Lucy, weighing 3.35 kg. The third stage progressed without any complications. Small vulval lacerations were left unsutured and Annabel and her baby were transferred to the postnatal area and went home the next morning. Annabel was so pleased with her labour and the care she had received that she and Jim sent a letter of thanks and praise to the Head of Midwifery, stating how much she had enjoyed and benefited from the aromatherapy.

Chapter 7

Essential Oils for Maternity Care

This chapter profiles 20 essential oils that are considered suitable for use in maternity care. Most are safe to use throughout pregnancy, labour and the puerperium, except two – clary sage and jasmine – which should only be used from term (from 37 weeks gestation) and one other – rose – which should only be used from the mid-third trimester (about 34 weeks). One essential oil, tea tree, is considered inappropriate for labour.

There are several other essential oils which are safe to use at this time, but which have not been included in this book. In clinical practice, it is wise to use only a small selection of versatile essential oils so that the midwife, doula or other care provider can become familiar with the indications, contraindications and precautions for each essential oil. This practice also prevents wastage from oxidisation of those essential oils which are less frequently used (see Chapters 2 and 3).

The following essential oil profiles provide a summary of the chemistry and the other essential oils with which they will blend well, from an aromatic perspective. There is direct application to maternity care practice in the indications, contraindications and precautions. The profiles also include the physiological and psychological effects which the oils have been reported to have and a brief acknowledgement of contemporary research findings where available (see also Chapter 3 and Table 7.1).

The charts are intended as a quick reference for use in clinical practice and can be cross-referenced to Chapter 6 on the use of aromatherapy in pregnancy and childbirth. A brief summary of carrier oils is also given here. The oils which have been included as suitable for maternity use are:

- bergamot
- black pepper
- chamomile, Roman
- clary sage (not pregnancy)
- cypress
- lavender
- lime
- mandarin/tangerine
- neroli
- orange, sweet

- eucalyptus
- frankincense
- geranium
- grapefruit
- jasmine (not pregnancy)

- peppermint
- rose (from 34 weeks gestation)
- spearmint
- tea tree (not labour)
- ylang ylang

Bergamot (*Citrus aurantium/ bergamia*) – fruit oil

Chemistry	α-pinene, β-pinene, mycrene, limonene, α-bergaptene, β-bisabolene, linalool, linalyl acetate, nerol, neryl acetate, geraniol, geraniol acetate, α-terpineol; furanocoumarins – bergapten (5-methoxypsoralen)
Blends well with	Black pepper, chamomile, clary sage, cypress, eucalyptus, frankincense, geranium, grapefruit, jasmine, lavender, lime, mandarin/tangerine, neroli, orange (sweet), peppermint, rose, spearmint, tea tree, ylang ylang NB An excellent oil to add to any other blend but the gentle aroma can be overpowered by stronger ones, so the proportion of bergamot may need to be higher than that of other essential oils
Reported effects	Antiseptic, antibacterial, antiviral, antifungal Analgesic Anticoagulant (mild) Antidepressant Antispasmodic Digestive aid Hypotensive Sedative
Indications	**Pregnancy** Relaxation – to ease fear, anxiety, stress Uplifting, mood enhancing Constipation, nausea, vomiting, flatulence, loss of appetite May be useful for skin conditions (e.g. pruritus from striae gravidarum) Pain relief – backache, headache, carpal tunnel syndrome, etc. Mild to moderate hypertension Insomnia, fatigue As compress over kidney region if there is urinary tract infection (with antibiotics)

Labour
Pain relief (indirect effect)
Facial spray to refresh
Relief of stress, anxiety, fear, tension
Nausea, vomiting

Postnatal
Aids emotional recovery from birth, prevention of postnatal 'blues', depression
Aids sleep
Constipation, nausea
Wound healing (direct application in dilution)
Prevention of infection

Contraindications and precautions	Avoid in women allergic to citrus fruit
	Mild skin irritation may occur if used neat on skin in susceptible women
	Furanocoumarins may cause photosensitivity (moderate, theoretical, dose-dependent risk) – avoid exposure of skin to direct sunlight for at least 12 hours – or use furanocoumarin-free
	Avoid with anticoagulants or drugs with similar action
	Avoid with vaginal bleeding (theoretical risk)
	Store in refrigerator to avoid oxidisation; shelf life 3–6 months; discard old or oxidised oil
	Occasionally adulterated with synthetic chemical constituents – purchase from reputable supplier
Evidence base	Psychological effects – mood enhancing, stress-reducing (Navarra *et al.* 2015)
	Reduces anxiety (Bagetta *et al.* 2010; Chang and Shen 2011; Ni *et al.* 2013)
	Less effective with raised BMI (Saiyudthong and Marsden 2011)
	May be anti-infective and wound healing (Cosentino *et al.* 2014; Nisticò *et al.* 2015)
	Antimicrobial (Laird and Phillips 2012)
	May be anti-ageing (Liu, Lin and Chang 2013)

Black pepper (*Piper nigrum*) – spice oil

Chemistry	Terpenoid hydrocarbons, α-pinene, β-pinene, δ-3 carene, limonene, β-caryophyllene, α-phellandrene, β-phellandrene, sabine
Blends well with	Bergamot, chamomile, clary sage, cypress, eucalyptus, frankincense, geranium, grapefruit, jasmine, lavender, lime, mandarin/tangerine, neroli, orange (sweet), peppermint, rose, spearmint, tea tree, ylang ylang
	A very distinctive aroma which will not suit all women but when used in minute amounts can be very therapeutically effective; best to use only 1–2 drops maximum in a blend
Reported effects	Analgesic – very strong
	Digestive stimulant, anti-emetic
	Antibacterial, antifungal
	Expectorant, anticatarrhal
	Febrifuge, rubefacient, vasodilatory
Indications	**Pregnancy**
	Pain relief (e.g. backache, sciatica, symphysis pubis pain, groin and ligament pain, neck ache, shoulder pain, headache, other muscular discomforts)
	Oedema, carpal tunnel syndrome
	Constipation, diarrhoea, nausea (caution due to strong aroma), heartburn, indigestion, hypersalivation, poor appetite, flatulence
	Sinusitis, colds, influenza, respiratory infections
	May aid smoking cessation in combination with counseling, etc.
	Mild to moderate hypertension
	Labour
	Excellent analgesia for first-stage labour
	Warming for feet in prolonged labour
	Nausea (caution)
	Postnatal
	Pain relief (e.g. post-epidural neck and back pain, post-Caesarean pain, headache, muscular discomfort)
	Constipation, nausea (caution), flatulence, diarrhoea, poor appetite
Contraindications and precautions	Mild phototoxicity risk, possibly exacerbated when used with other oils which cause photosensitivity, such as citrus oils
	Can be irritating to skin and eyes
	Strong aroma makes it a specific oil to avoid with homeopathic remedies
	Caution with diabetic women with poorly controlled blood glucose

Evidence base	Pain relief (neck ache) (Ou *et al.* 2014)
	Effective against persistent *Staph. aureus* (Lee *et al.* 2014a)
	May ease nicotine withdrawal (Cordell and Buckle 2013; Kitikannakorn *et al.* 2013)
	Inhalation may aid swallowing reflex (Ebihara *et al.* 2006)
	May have a part to play in reducing blood sugar (type 2 diabetes) and blood pressure (Oboh *et al.* 2013)
	Topical use may aid intravenous needle insertion (Kristiniak *et al.* 2012)

Chamomile, Roman (*Chamaemelum nobile/anthemis nobilis*) – flower oil

Chemistry	α-pinene, α-terpinene, α–thujene, borneol, azulene, (chamazulene produced on extraction), pinocarveol, pinocarvone, isoamyl angelate, camphene, β-myrcene, β-pinene, butyrate esthers, apigenin-7-glucoside, α-bisabolol, farnesene
Blends well with	Bergamot, clary sage, cypress, eucalyptus, frankincense, geranium, grapefruit, jasmine, lavender, lime, mandarin/tangerine, neroli, orange (sweet), peppermint, rose, spearmint, tea tree, ylang ylang
	Strong, distinctive aroma which can be suppressed with citrus oils or other sharp-smelling oils such as eucalyptus
Reported effects	Analgesic
	Antiseptic, antibacterial, antifungal, antiviral
	Anticoagulant (mild)
	Anti-inflammatory, wound healing (direct application in dilution)
	Anti-oxidant
	Antispasmodic
	Calming, sedating
	Digestive stimulant, anti-emetic
Contraindications and precautions	Use well-diluted on skin – risk of contact dermatitis (Maddocks-Jennings 2004)
	(Nipple irritation has previously been reported from use of a commercial nipple protection ointment containing Roman chamomile (McGeorge and Steele 1991))

Indications	**Pregnancy** Pain relief for physical discomforts – backache, neck ache, sciatica Prevention of infection Constipation, nausea, vomiting, flatulence, irritable bowel syndrome Insomnia, tiredness, fatigue Anxiety, tension Skin conditions (e.g. eczema), with caution, using no more than 1% blend **Labour** Pain relief Regulate contractions Tiredness, anxiety, fear **Postnatal** Wound healing (direct application in dilution) – Caesarean, episiotomy, sore nipples (caution) Constipation, anti-emetic, diarrhoea, irritable bowel syndrome Tiredness, anxiety, stress
Evidence base	Anti-oxidant (Agatonovic-Kustrin *et al.* 2015) Analgesic, relieves oedema (Tomić *et al.* 2014) Eases migraine headache (Zargaran *et al.* 2014) Antifungal (Jamalian *et al.* 2012) May cause allergic reactions (Maddocks-Jennings 2004) Calming, sedating, reduced alertness (Moss *et al.* 2006) Wound healing (Woollard,Tatham and Barker 2007)

Clary sage (*Salvia sclarea*) – leaf and flower oil

Chemistry	Linalool, linalyl acetate, mycrene, phellandrene, pinene, β-caryophyllene, sclareol, 1.8 cineole, germacrene D; thought to contain over 250 constituents
Blends well with	Bergamot, chamomile, cypress, eucalyptus, frankincense, geranium, grapefruit, jasmine, lavender, lime, mandarin/tangerine, neroli, orange (sweet), peppermint, rose, spearmint, tea tree, ylang ylang Strong medicinal aroma which not all women like; best to use blend in which clary sage constitutes a small proportion of the overall aroma

Reported effects	Analgesic (strong) Antibacterial, antifungal, antiviral Antispasmodic Antidepressant, euphoric 'Oestrogenic' – possibly due to sclareol content – emmenagoguic, uterotonic Sedative Expectorant
Indications	**Pregnancy** ABSOLUTELY NONE – DO NOT USE BEFORE 37 WEEKS **Labour** Pain relief in labour (*avoid* if contractions well established) Induction, acceleration after 37 weeks only Retained placenta (fundal compress, with caution) Anxiety, fear, tension (avoid if contractions well established) **Postnatal** Postnatal 'blues', depression Pain relief Respiratory infections, sinus congestion Mild to moderate hypertension
Contraindications and precautions	DO NOT USE UNTIL TERM – CONSIDER CLARY SAGE AS 'NATURE'S SYNTOCINON' Avoid if labour is well established – may cause hypertonic uterine action and fetal distress Clary sage is frequently over-used or abused: anecdotal reports have revealed fetal distress, which appears to be dose-dependent and gestation-dependent Advise women not to self-administer clary sage; question women in preterm labour about possible self-administration Not to be used neat on the abdomen; not to be used in a vaporiser Not to be used for retained products of conception – may precipitate secondary postpartum haemorrhage Care in early puerperium when lochia are heavy Midwives and other care providers should take care when menstruating – may cause menorrhagia with prolonged exposure; not to be used by midwives who are attempting to conceive, undergoing fertility treatment, or who are pregnant or breastfeeding Avoid alcohol – may potentiate sedative properties May cause mild skin irritation May cause headache or drowsiness in high doses; midwives should take care when driving immediately after using clary sage with labouring women May be adulterated with other substances containing linalool or linalyl acetate, either natural or synthetic

NB Renowned essential oil authorities, Tisserand and Young (2014) claim that there is no reason to avoid clary sage, since any emmenagoguic, oestrogen-like sclareol content appears only in the absolute and not in the essential oil. However, the maternity-specific precautions listed here are from many years of this author's clinical experience and the increasing tendency of pregnant women to purchase clary sage oil as a natural means of inducing labour. Numerous anecdotal reports of hypertonic uterine contractions at term, apparently idiopathic preterm labour, fetal distress and even stillbirth have been reported to this author. Reports of adverse effects on staff have included drowsiness, lethargy, loss of concentration and – significantly – menorrhagia in midwives caring for women using clary sage in labour. In fairness, most adverse effects appear to arise from injudicious use and misguided over-use, from lack of knowledge amongst both professionals and mothers, of the correct dosage, duration and frequency of use and other relevant precautions.

Evidence base	Aids progress in labour (Burns *et al.* 2000) Antidepressant, reduces cortisol and 5-HT in post-menopausal women (Lee, Cho and Kang 2014b; Yang *et al.* 2014) Reduces blood pressure, stress (Seol *et al.* 2013) Relieves dysmenorrhoea (Ou *et al.* 2012) Antidepressant (Seol *et al.* 2010)

Cypress (*Cupressus sempervirens*) – leaf oil

Chemistry	α-pinene, cedrol, sabinol, terpenyl acetate, camphene, limonene, β-mycrene, β-pinene, sabinene, guaiol, guaiazulene, chamazulene, cadalene, elemol, β-eudesmol
Blends well with	Bergamot, chamomile, clary sage, eucalyptus, frankincense, geranium, grapefruit, jasmine, lavender, lime, mandarin/tangerine, neroli, orange (sweet), peppermint, rose, spearmint, tea tree, ylang ylang Distinctive, somewhat masculine and sharp aroma, which can be very pleasant when used in synergistic blend with more 'rounded' aromas such as rose, spearmint, ylang ylang
Reported effects	Antibacterial, antifungal Antispasmodic Astringent; phlebotonic, vasoconstrictive Calming Diuretic Mucus stimulant, expectorant, decongestant

Indications	**Pregnancy** Leg cramps, cellulitis Cystitis (non-infective) Haemorrhoids, varicosities Oedema, carpal tunnel syndrome Sinus congestion, colds, coughs Relaxing, calming, eases nervous tension, stress relief Constipation, flatulence, intestinal cramps **Labour** Oedema, pelvic congestion Pain relief, eases tension, fear, anxiety Generally mood stimulating **Postnatal** Oedema, carpal tunnel syndrome; leg cramps Cystitis (non-infective) Sinus congestion; colds, coughs Relaxing, calming Tiredness, fatigue Constipation, flatulence, intestinal cramps Haemorrhoids, varicosities Wound healing
Contraindications and precautions	Caution in hypertensive women due to vasoconstriction Possible skin sensitisation if the essential oil has oxidised – avoid neat application Store in refrigerator to avoid premature oxidisation
Evidence base	Antimicrobial (Arjouni *et al.* 2011; Selim *et al.* 2014) May have antidiabetic effect (Asgary *et al.* 2013) Possible CNS depressant (Umezu 2012)

Eucalyptus (*Eucalyptus globulus*) – leaf oil

Chemistry	1.8 cineole (possibly up to 80%), α-pinene, limonene, α-terpineol, β-pinene, globulol, pinocarveol, camphene, fenchene, phellandrene; up to 250 constituents
Blends well with	Bergamot, chamomile, clary sage, cypress, frankincense, geranium, grapefruit, jasmine, lavender, lime, mandarin/tangerine, neroli, orange (sweet), peppermint, rose, spearmint, tea tree, ylang ylang Distinctive aroma which blends well with all oils in the profiles here, but which some women may prefer in small proportions, balanced by other oils

Reported effects	Anti-inflammatory Analgesic – especially muscular Antibacterial, antiseptic Anti-oxidant Expectorant, decongestant Increases alertness Rubefacient, may reduce pyrexia
Indications	**Pregnancy** Respiratory conditions – sinusitis, colds, influenza, bronchitis Pain relief – backache, shoulder pain, neck ache, headache Urinary tract infection, pyrexia Balance to sedative oils **Labour** Pain relief General relaxation Pyrexia Balance to sedative oils **Postnatal** Respiratory conditions – sinusitis, colds, influenza, bronchitis Pain relief – backache, shoulder pain, neck ache, headache Prevention of infection Balance to sedative oils
Contraindications and precautions	Avoid strong concentrations to prevent skin or respiratory tract irritation Do not use in women with asthma Avoid in combination with homeopathic remedies; do not store with homeopathic remedies Do not take internally Keep out of the reach of children – has been known to cause CNS and respiratory problems (Tisserand and Young 2014). These authorities cite several incidents of children being severely adversely affected by dermal administration of oil blends containing eucalyptus for treatment of head lice and pruritis. However, they do not concur with the original German Commission E contraindications, which they believe were based on 1.8 cineole-rich eucalyptus oil (Blumenthal et al. 2000). Eucalyptus poisoning from internal administration has been largely witnessed in Australia as a result of children ingesting the oil: Australia now uses child-resistant containers for eucalyptus essential oil. The cardinal signs of eucalyptus poisoning are CNS depression, abnormal respiration and pin-point pupils but may also include epigastric pain, nausea, vomiting, headaches, muscle weakness, slurred speech, clammy skin and cold sweats, tachycardia, vertigo, drowsiness, coma and loss of consciousness (see Chapter 4 for safety information).

Evidence base	Antimicrobial (Karbach *et al.* 2015)
	May be antitubercular (Rehman, Ali and Khan 2014)
	Mosquito repellent (Ramos Alvarenga *et al.* 2014)
	Antifungal (Ben Hassine *et al.* 2012)
	Antibacterial, antiviral (Elaissi *et al.* 2012)
	May increase alertness, possibly due to stimulation of trigeminal nerve (Buchbauer 1996)
	Mucolytic, anti-inflammatory in sinusitis (Kehrl, Sommermann and Dethlefsen 2004)
	Peripheral antinociceptive action and dose-related central analgesic (Silva *et al.* 2003)

Frankincense/olibanum (*Boswellia carteri/sacra*) – gum resin oil

Chemistry	α-pinene, α-phellandrene, β-cymene, β-pinene, β-caryophyllene α-thujene, β-ocimene, limonene, borneol, farnesol, terpinen-4-ol, sabinene, mycrene, camphene, octanol acetate, octyl acetate, linalool, 1.8 cineole, verticilla-4(20),7,11,triene (Mertens, Buettner and Kirchoff 2009)
Blends well with	Bergamot, chamomile, clary sage, cypress, eucalyptus, geranium, grapefruit, jasmine, lavender, lime, mandarin/tangerine, neroli, orange (sweet), peppermint, rose, spearmint, tea tree, ylang ylang
	Distinctive aroma which can be used on its own or in combination with citrus oils to suppress the slightly medicinal aroma
Reported effects	Analgesic
	Antiseptic, antibacterial, antifungal, antiviral
	Calming yet mentally stimulating
	Decongestant, expectorant
Indications	**Pregnancy**
	Expectorant for colds, influenza, sinus congestion
	Relaxation, balancing of emotions – anxiety, stress, tension, mild depression
	Tiredness, fatigue
	Useful for extreme fear (e.g. prior to phlebotomy)
	May be useful for irritable bowel syndrome
	Labour
	Pain relief
	Anxiety, tension
	Excellent for transition stage – 'the ultimate calmer'
	Also good for women prior to elective Caesarean section as pre-medication

	Postnatal Depression, postnatal 'blues' Tiredness, fatigue, stress, anxiety Respiratory conditions – sinus congestion, colds, influenza
Contraindications and precautions	Skin sensitivity may occur if the oil has oxidised – avoid old oils May be wise to avoid in asthmatic women who respond adversely to strong odours Store in refrigerator to avoid oxidisation Ensure purity – frankincense trees are considered a threatened species, plus loss of skills in harvesting the resin from beneath the bark has increased price and led to the possibility of adulteration with other substances
Evidence base	Analgesic (Al-Harrassi *et al.* 2014) Anti-inflammatory (Mostafa *et al.* 2015; Siddiqui 2011) May have antitumoral effects (Ni *et al.* 2012; Suhail *et al.* 2011) May help in irritable bowel syndrome (Alyssa Parian 2015; Langhorst *et al.* 2015)

Geranium (*Pelargonium graveolens*) – leaf oil

Chemistry	Citronellol, geraniol, linalool, citronellyl acetate, geranyl acetate, *iso*-menthone, linalyl acetate, β-caryophyllene, neral, geranial, citronellal, menthone
Blends well with	Bergamot, chamomile, clary sage, cypress, eucalyptus, frankincense, grapefruit, jasmine, lavender, lime, mandarin/tangerine, neroli, orange (sweet), peppermint, rose, spearmint, tea tree, ylang ylang Very floral aroma loved by many women
Reported effects	Analgesic Antibacterial, antifungal Anti-inflammatory Astringent, wound healing (direct application), aids circulation Possibly diuretic Uplifting, calming, reduces anxiety, nervous tension, agitation Balances mood swings Geranium oil is thought to be a balancer – of hormones, mood and general wellbeing. However, in the experience of this author, some women may react with an exacerbation of the presenting symptoms rather than an inhibition. This appears to be dose-dependent in the main but may also be related to the specific presentation of the condition at any given time, particularly with psycho-emotional issues.

Indications	**Pregnancy** Relaxation, anxiety, fear, mood swings Pain relief – backache, neck ache, leg cramps Oedema, carpal tunnel syndrome Varicosities, haemorrhoids Wound healing (direct application in dilution) Prevention of infection **Labour** Pain relief Relaxation, fear, anxiety, calming, mood variations May have indirect effect on labour progress through relaxation effect **Postnatal** Infections Relaxation, general wellbeing Postnatal 'blues', mood swings, anxiety, tension, recovery from birth Oedema, carpal tunnel syndrome Varicosities, haemorrhoids Wound healing (direct application in dilution)
Contraindications and precautions	May be adulterated with cheaper, similar-smelling oils, so purchase from reputable suppliers Caution with hypertensive women due to astringent effect which may cause vasoconstriction Can cause skin irritation in susceptible women Beware effect on women prone to hayfever and asthma triggered by flower pollen – psychosomatic effect Can cause nausea in strong dilutions in susceptible women Avoid oral use in diabetic women on medication – may interact, lead to hypoglycaemia (theoretical risk)
Evidence base	Antibacterial (Sienkiewicz *et al.* 2014) Anti-inflammatory (Boukhatem *et al.* 2013) Reduced oedema in mice (Maruyama *et al.* 2006) May be antidiabetic (Boukhris *et al.* 2012) Antifungal (Azimi *et al.* 2011) Analgesic, antineuralgic (Greenway *et al.* 2003) Reduces fear and anxiety in first-stage labour (Rashidi Fakari *et al.* 2015)

Grapefruit (*Citrus x paradisi*) – fruit oil

Chemistry	Limonene, geraniol, citronellal, neral, β-myrcene, α-pinene, sabinene, bergapten, bergamottin
Blends well with	Bergamot, chamomile, clary sage, cypress, eucalyptus, frankincense, geranium, jasmine, lavender, lime, mandarin/tangerine, neroli, orange (sweet), peppermint, rose, spearmint, tea tree, ylang ylang NB An excellent oil to add to any other blend but gentle aroma can be overpowered by stronger ones, so proportion of grapefruit in a blend may need to be higher than that of other essential oils
Reported effects	Analgesic (mild) Anti-inflammatory Antiseptic, antibacterial, antiviral, antifungal Calming, refreshing, uplifting (mood) Gastric stimulant Immunostimulant Possibly diuretic, improves lymphatic flow Tonic, hypotensive
Indications	**Pregnancy** Stress, anxiety, depression, mood swings, tension Nausea, vomiting, pica, constipation, loss of appetite, hypersalivation Headaches, colds, influenza Pain relief (indirect) Mild to moderate hypertension Prevention of infection Compress over kidney region for urinary tract infection (with antibiotics) Oedema, carpal tunnel syndrome **Labour** Fear, anxiety, tension, stress Pain relief (indirect) General wellbeing, relaxation Mild to moderate hypertension **Postnatal** Prevention of infection General wellbeing, emotional calming, relaxation Uplifting to reduce postnatal 'blues' Stress, anxiety, fatigue, insomnia Oedema, carpal tunnel syndrome Constipation, flatulence, irritable bowel syndrome, nausea Wound healing (direct application in dilution) Reputed to aid weight loss

Contraindications and precautions	Avoid in women allergic to citrus fruit
	Photosensitivity – avoid exposure of skin to direct sunlight for 12 hours
	May cause skin irritation in strong doses
	Avoid with anticoagulants or drugs with similar action
	Avoid with vaginal bleeding (theoretical)
	Store in refrigerator to avoid oxidisation; shelf life 3–6 months
	Avoid oral use – grapefruit juice is contraindicated with many medications and although the essential oil does not contain as many of the chemicals responsible for any potential interaction, there is a slight possibility
Evidence base	May aid weight loss (Haze *et al.* 2010; Shen *et al.* 2005)
	Decreases gastric nerve activity, blood pressure, heat production (Nagai *et al.* 2014)

Jasmine (*Jasminum officinale/ grandifolium*) – flower oil

Chemistry	Benzyl acetate, linalool, benzyl alcohol, methyl jasmonate, indole, benzyl benzoate, *cis*-jasmone, geraniol, methyl anthranilate, farnesol, *cis*-3-hexenyl benzoate, eugenol, nerol, benzoic acid, benzaldehyde, γ-terpineol, nerolidol, isophytol, phytol
Blends well with	Bergamot, chamomile, clary sage, cypress, eucalyptus, frankincense, geranium, grapefruit, lavender, lime, mandarin/tangerine, neroli, orange (sweet), peppermint, rose, spearmint, tea tree, ylang ylang
	Heavy, somewhat cloying aroma which can be overpowering if used in high doses
Reported effects	Analgesic
	Antibacterial, antifungal, antiviral
	Antispasmodic
	Aphrodisiac, calming, relaxing
	Conversely, may be stimulating (Heuberger and Ilmberger 2010)
	Emmenagoguic, uterotonic
	Pain relieving
Indications	**Pregnancy**
	DO NOT USE IN PREGNANCY BEFORE 37 WEEKS GESTATION
	Calming, relaxation, fear of birth, preparation for birth
	Birth 'priming' in regular treatments from 37 weeks gestation

Labour

General wellbeing, relaxation, anxiety, stress, fear, tension, tiredness, insomnia

Pain relief, discomfort

Enhances uterine action, induction and acceleration of labour, retained placenta

Postnatal

After pains – with care and avoid if retained products

General wellbeing and relaxation, recovery from birth

Stress, 'blues', depression, low mood, improve confidence in mothering

Backache, general aches and pains

May aid lactation although some early papers suggest inhibits lactation (Abraham, Devi and Sheela 1979; Shrivastav et al.1988)

Contraindications and precautions	DO NOT USE IN PREGNANCY UNTIL 37 WEEKS – possibly emmenagoguic due to ketone content Aroma may be overpowering, nauseating and may induce narcosis or headache, especially in high doses May be adulterated – purchase from reputable company to ensure purity Beware effect on women prone to hayfever and asthma triggered by flower pollen – psychosomatic effect May cause skin irritation. Tisserand and Young (2014) suggest that this risk is slightly higher in people of Asian origin than in those of black or Caucasian origin, although they admit that the issue of adulteration of this costly oil may have been responsible for some cases of alleged allergic reactions
Evidence base	Sedative, relaxing (Kuroda et al. 2005) Improves concentration and hand–eye coordination in sport (Hirsch et al. 2007b) Stimulating, mood uplifting (Hongratanaworakit 2010) Effective against E. coli (Rath et al. 2008) Possible stimulating effect (Heuberger and Ilmberger 2010; Lis-Balchin, Hart and Wan Hang Lo 2002) May lower prolactin, inhibiting lactation (Finny et al. 2015)

Lavender, common (*Lavandula angustifolia/officinalis*) – flower oil

Chemistry	Linalyl acetate, linalool, terpinenol, cineole, β-caryophyllene, farnascene, coumarin, geranyl acetate, camphor
Blends well with	Bergamot, chamomile, clary sage, cypress, eucalyptus, frankincense, geranium, grapefruit, jasmine, lime, mandarin/tangerine, neroli, orange (sweet), peppermint, rose, spearmint, tea tree, ylang ylang Distinctive aroma loved by many women, although young mothers may associate it with the elderly
Reported effects	Analgesic Antibacterial, mildly antiviral Anti-inflammatory Carminative, digestive Expectorant, decongestant Relaxing; sedative, calming Hypotensive Muscle relaxant, antispasmodic
Indications	**Pregnancy** General wellbeing and relaxation Stress, anxiety, tension, fear Fatigue and insomnia Headaches and migraine, backache, sciatica, symphysis pubis pain, shoulder and neck pain Oedema, carpal tunnel syndrome Mild to moderate hypertension (*avoid* in fulminating pre-eclampsia) Colds and influenza, sinus congestion Constipation, flatulence, nausea (low doses) **Labour** Pain relief Anxiety, fear, tension, panic, tiredness Natural induction, augments uterine action, retained placenta (mild effect) General wellbeing and relaxation

Postnatal
Stress, anxiety, tension, fear; general relaxation
Insomnia; tiredness
Headaches and migraine, backache,
sciatica, symphysis pubis pain
Oedema, carpal tunnel syndrome
Post-Caesarean recovery – pain relief, gastric stimulation,
wound healing (direct application in dilution)
Episiotomy pain and wound healing (direct application in water,
in dilution; do not use on sanitary towel or neat on suture line)
Mild to moderate hypertension
Colds, influenza, sinus congestion
Constipation, flatulence, nausea (low doses)

Contraindications and precautions

Can cause skin irritation in susceptible women
or with excessively strong concentrations
Caution if postural/supine hypotension;
also with epidural anaesthesia
Can have sedative effect or cause loss of concentration in staff
Beware effect on women prone to hayfever and asthma
triggered by flower pollen – psychosomatic effect
Caution when using for episiotomy pain and wound
healing – use very dilute doses in water, dry area
thoroughly after administration to aid wound healing
Gynaecomastia has been reported in pre-pubertal
boys exposed to high doses of lavender oil or
essence (Diaz et al. 2015; Henley et al. 2007)

Evidence base

Relaxing, anxiolytic (de Souza et al. 2015; Lehrner et al. 2005;
Perry et al. 2012; Takahashi et al. 2014; Zabirunnisa et al. 2014)
Analgesic, including post-operatively (general)
(Bagheri-Nesami et al. 2014; Kim et al. 2006; Olapour
et al. 2013; Raisi Dehkordi et al. 2014)
Lavender massage reduces pain in labour and duration of first
and second stage (Abbaspoor and Mohammadkhani 2013)
Reduces post-Caesarean pain (Lillehei and
Halcon 2014; Olapour et al. 2013)
Aids sleep (Chen and Chen 2015; Lytle, Mwatha
and Davis 2014; Sheikhan et al. 2012)
Wound healing (Kim et al. 2007)
Useful for episiotomy healing and pain (Kim et al. 2006, 2007;
Sheikhan et al. 2012; Soltani et al. 2013; Vakilian et al. 2011)
Reduces need for post-operative analgesia
(Irmak Sapmaz et al. 2015)
May ease pain in renal colic (Sayorwan et al. 2012)
Reduces blood pressure (Tanida et al. 2006)

Lime (*Citrus aurantium*) – fruit oil

Chemistry	Citral, β-pinene, γ-terpinene, ρ-cymene, terpinen-4-ol, α-terpineol, δ-limonene, linalool, α-bergamotene, camphene, sabinene
Blends well with	Bergamot, chamomile, clary sage, cypress, eucalyptus, frankincense, geranium, grapefruit, jasmine, lavender, mandarin/tangerine, neroli, orange (sweet), peppermint, rose, spearmint, tea tree, ylang ylang Sharp aroma similar to Starburst® sweets
Reported effects	Improves alertness, concentration Reduces blood pressure, astringent Uplifting, calming, relaxing Skin care Anti-emetic Anti-inflammatory Antispasmodic Antipyrexial Immune system balancer May have hepatic effect Anticoagulant (mild)
Indications	**Pregnancy** Relaxation, stress, anxiety, mild depression Insomnia, fatigue Nausea, vomiting, pica, constipation, diarrhoea, heartburn, poor appetite, irritable bowel syndrome Varicosities, haemorrhoids Mild to moderate hypertension Facial acne (facial spray) Maintain concentration and energy at work **Labour** Pain relief General wellbeing, anxiety, fear, stress, tension, uplifting and stimulating Nausea, vomiting Pelvic congestion **Postnatal** General wellbeing, relaxation, stress, anxiety, tension Postnatal 'blues' and mild depression, insomnia, tiredness Nausea, vomiting, post-Caesarean Irritable bowel syndrome Prevention of infection, enhances immune system

Contraindications and precautions	Avoid in women allergic to citrus fruit Avoid exposure of skin to direct sunlight for at least two hours Caution with hypertensive women due to astringent effect Avoid with anticoagulants or drugs with similar action Avoid with vaginal bleeding (theoretical) Store in refrigerator to avoid oxidisation; shelf life 3–6 months
Evidence base	Improves alertness (Heuberger *et al.* 2001) Reduces systolic blood pressure (Saiyudthong *et al.* 2009) Antispasmodic (Spadaro *et al.* 2012) May aid weight loss (Asnaashari *et al.* 2010) Antibacterial (Aibinu *et al.* 2006)

Mandarin/tangerine (*Citrus reticulata*) – fruit oil

Chemistry	Limonene, linalool, thymol, anthranilates (may cause 'fishy' odour when oxidised) These two essential oils are very similar in chemical make-up and are often classed together. However, true tangerine contains esters, while true mandarin does not.
Blends well with	Bergamot, black pepper, chamomile, clary sage, cypress, eucalyptus, frankincense, geranium, grapefruit, jasmine, lavender, lime, neroli, orange (sweet), peppermint, rose, spearmint, tea tree, ylang ylang The aroma is more 'rounded' or 'creamy' than some other citrus oils such as lime or grapefruit and blends well with any of the oils in the profiles contained here.
Reported effects	Diuretic, reduces oedema Aids weight loss Skin conditions Relaxing, calming, uplifting Antifungal, antibacterial Antispasmodic

Indications	**Pregnancy** Relaxation, stress, fear, anxiety, insomnia, restlessness, fatigue Striae gravidarum, facial acne Constipation, colic, diarrhoea, irritable bowel syndrome Prevent/treat minor infections, especially skin conditions **Labour** Relaxation, stress, fear, anxiety Pain relief (indirect) **Postnatal** Relaxation, stress, fear, anxiety, insomnia, restlessness, fatigue Constipation, colic, diarrhoea, irritable bowel syndrome Prevent/treat minor infections, especially minor skin conditions
Contraindications and precautions	Avoid in women allergic to citrus fruit Avoid exposure of skin to direct sunlight for at least two hours (although the furocoumarin content is less than that of bergamot) Avoid with anticoagulants or drugs with similar action Caution in women with eczema, psoriasis Avoid with vaginal bleeding (theoretical risk) Store in refrigerator to avoid oxidisation; shelf life 3–6 months; discard old or oxidised oils
Evidence base	Antimicrobial action affected by proportion of linalool in oils from different sources (Herman, Tambor and Herman 2015) Anxiolytic effect (de Sousa *et al.* 2015) No other direct clinical or *in vitro* research evidence was found, despite an extensive literature search, although some studies investigating 'citrus' essential oils in general include mandarin (also sometimes known as tangerine). Non-clinical research focuses on chemical constituents, particularly in relation to growth, harvesting and the food industry.

Neroli (*Citrus aurantium; Neroli bigarade*) – orange blossom – flower oil

Chemistry	Linalyl acetate, limonene, linalool, farnesol, nerolidol, geraniol, α-terpineol, indol, geranyl acetate, neryl acetate, methyl anthranilate, benzyl acetate, jasmine, limonene, camphene, α-pinene, β-pinene, β-ocimene
Blends well with	Bergamot, chamomile, clary sage, cypress, eucalyptus, frankincense, geranium, grapefruit, jasmine, lavender, lime, mandarin/tangerine, orange (sweet), peppermint, rose, spearmint, tea tree, ylang ylang Subtle aroma which takes time to warm up and become noticeable

Reported effects	Antibacterial, antiviral Sedative, relaxing, relieves anxiety Hypotensive Antispasmodic Aphrodisiac Wound healing
Indications	**Pregnancy** Anxiety, fear, depression, general relaxation and wellbeing Nausea and vomiting, constipation, diarrhoea, irritable bowel syndrome Relationship issues, loss of libido Cramps – muscular, intestinal Insomnia, tiredness, fatigue Skin care, theoretical effect on reducing striae gravidarum Wound healing, immunity stimulant **Labour** Generally mood uplifting Reduces anxiety, fear Relieves nausea, vomiting Indirectly aids pain relief May aid progress in labour **Postnatal** Prevention/treatment of postnatal 'blues'/depression General wellbeing, relaxation, relief of anxiety Tiredness, insomnia, fatigue Constipation, post-Caesarean paralytic ileus, diarrhoea, nausea, vomiting, flatulence
Contraindications and precautions	Avoid in women allergic to citrus fruit Avoid exposure of skin to direct sunlight for at least two hours Avoid with anticoagulants or drugs with similar action Avoid with vaginal bleeding (theoretical) Store in refrigerator to avoid oxidisation; shelf life 3–6 months Beware effect on women prone to hayfever and asthma triggered by flower pollen – psychosomatic effect
Evidence base	Analgesic, anti-inflammatory (Khodabakhsh, Shafaroodi and Asgarpanah 2015) Reduces first-stage anxiety (Namazi *et al.* 2014a) Aids pain relief in labour (Namazi 2014b) Possibly anti-convulsant (Azanchi, Shafaroodi and Asgarpanah 2014) Reduces cortisol, blood pressure (Choi *et al.* 2014; Kim *et al.* 2012)

Orange, sweet (*Citrus sinensis*) – fruit oil

Chemistry	Limonene, camphene, α-pinene, myrcene, sabinene, citral, octanal, decanal, neryl acetate, 1.8 cineole, furanocoumarins, β-carvone, α-ionone, fenchol, terpineol, linalool, nerol
Blends well with	Bergamot, chamomile, clary sage, cypress, eucalyptus, frankincense, geranium, grapefruit, jasmine, lavender, mandarin, neroli, peppermint, rose, spearmint, tangerine, tea tree, ylang ylang Distinctive well-'rounded' aroma, which is considerably less sharp than other citrus oils such as grapefruit and lime
Reported effects	Analgesic Relaxing Antibacterial, antifungal, antiseptic Circulatory stimulant May aid smooth muscle contraction May stimulate lymphatic system May have beneficial effect on skin
Indications	**Pregnancy** Uplifting, relaxing, mood enhancing, stress, anxiety, fear Fatigue, insomnia Skin irritation, pruritus Oedema, carpal tunnel syndrome Nausea, vomiting, heartburn, constipation, diarrhoea, irritable bowel syndrome General wellbeing and pain relief (indirect) Anti-infective **Labour** Mood enhancing Reduces fear and tension General wellbeing and relaxation – may have indirect effect on labour progress Analgesic **Postnatal** Recovery from birth Relaxation, general wellbeing, postnatal 'blues' Insomnia, fatigue Constipation, flatulence, nausea, diarrhoea, irritable bowel syndrome 'After pains', general pain relief (indirect) Prevention of infection

Contraindications and precautions	Avoid in women allergic to citrus fruit Avoid exposure of skin to direct sunlight for at least two hours Avoid if skin itching Avoid with anticoagulants or drugs with similar action Avoid with vaginal bleeding (theoretical) Store in refrigerator to avoid oxidisation; shelf life 3–6 months; discard old or oxidised oils
Evidence base	Relaxing (Igarashi *et al.* 2014) Reduces anxiety, lifts mood (Faturi *et al.* 2010; Goes *et al.* 2012; Lehrner *et al.* 2005) Decreases autonomic arousal, enhances positive mood, de-stressing (Hongratanaworakit and Buchbauer 2007) Effective against MRSA and *Staph. aureus* (Muthaiyan *et al.* 2012)

Peppermint (*Mentha piperata*) – herb oil

Chemistry	Menthol, menthyl acetate, menthone, 1.8 cineole, limonene, menthofuran, phellandrene, β-pinene, β-caryophellene, terpineol-4-ol, β-pulegone, piperitone, isomenthol, pulegone
Blends well with	Bergamot, chamomile, clary sage, cypress, eucalyptus, frankincense, geranium, grapefruit, jasmine, lavender, lime, mandarin/tangerine, neroli, orange (sweet), rose, spearmint, tea tree, ylang ylang Sharp distinctive aroma
Reported effects	Antibacterial, antifungal Analgesic Decongestant Anti-emetic; aids digestion, colic; harmonises irritable bowel syndrome; reduces colonic motility Anti-inflammatory Antispasmodic Antipruritic Stimulating – cooling to skin Aids alertness Uplifting (mood)

Indications	**Pregnancy** Nausea, vomiting Heartburn, indigestion, irritable bowel syndrome, constipation, diarrhoea Muscular aches and pains, headaches, migraine General wellbeing, relaxation, stress, anxiety, fatigue, mood stimulating Colds, influenza, sinus congestion Skin irritation Oedema Tired, aching legs and feet **Labour** Pain relief Relaxation, mood uplifting, general wellbeing Nausea, vomiting May facilitate uterine action (very mild) **Postnatal** Nausea, constipation, diarrhoea, flatulence, heartburn, irritable bowel syndrome Recovery from birth Uplifting, mood enhancing Tiredness, fatigue Pain relief (mild) May aid wound healing
Contraindications and precautions	Avoid in women with cardiac disease, especially fibrillation and those on calcium antagonists Avoid in epileptics Do not use with, or store next to, homeopathic remedies (inactivates them) May cause skin irritation if used neat Can cause mucus membrane sensitivity – do not use *per vaginam* or *per rectum* May cause sleep disturbance in high doses – best not used for insomnia May be hepatotoxic or neurotoxic in large doses Avoid in women with G6PD (Tisserand and Young 2014) Contraindicated in babies and young children – has caused neonatal jaundice and may cause reflex apnoea (Tester-Dalderup 1980)

Evidence base	Antifungal (Samber *et al.* 2015)
	Analgesic (Davies, Harding and Baranowski 2002; Ou *et al.* 2014)
	Anti-emetic (Lua and Zakaria 2012; Stea, Beraudi and De Pasquale 2014)
	May ease post-Caesarean nausea (Lane *et al.* 2012)
	Reduces colonic spasm (Shavakhi *et al.* 2012)
	Reduces IBS symptoms (Cappello *et al.* 2007; Cash, Epstein and Shah 2015; Kearns *et al.* 2015)
	Inhibits intestinal smooth muscle spasm in IBS (mechanism of action) (Amato, Liota and Mulè 2014)
	Enhances concentration and memory (Moss *et al.* 2008)
	May be useful for hair loss (Oh *et al.* 2014)

Rose (*Rosa damascena* or *centifolia*) – flower oil

Chemistry	Phenyl ethanol, eugenol, citronellol, geraniol, nerol, farnesol, esters, rose oxide, limonene, myrcene, pinene
Blends well with	Bergamot, chamomile, clary sage, cypress, eucalyptus, frankincense, geranium, grapefruit, jasmine, lavender, lime, mandarin/tangerine, neroli, orange (sweet), peppermint, spearmint, tea tree, ylang ylang
	Subtle, feminine aroma which blends well with strong aromas such as lavender, black pepper and peppermint
Reported effects	Antibacterial, antifungal
	Analgesic
	Vasoconstrictive, astringent
	Cicatrisant
	Immunostimulant
	Anti-inflammatory
	Digestive
	Relaxing
	Antidepressant
	Aphrodisiac

Indications	**Pregnancy** DO NOT USE UNTIL 34 WEEKS GESTATION General wellbeing, relaxation Anxiety, depression, fear, tension Insomnia, fatigue, tiredness Constipation, nausea Pain relief – backache, neck pain, carpal tunnel syndrome, sciatica, pelvic pain, aching legs, etc. Relationship difficulties, loss of libido Skin conditions Prevention of infection May be useful for haemorrhoids due to vasoconstrictive effect **Labour** Pain relief Anxiety, fear, tension Uplifting, calming, relaxing May aid contractions **Postnatal** Postnatal 'blues', depression, stress, general relaxation, wellbeing Recovery from birth Eczema and other skin conditions, with caution, maximum 1% blend Pain relief Constipation, nausea, flatulence Sexual difficulties, loss of libido
Contraindications and precautions	Avoid until late third trimester (from 34 weeks gestation) due to possible mild emmenagoguic action Beware effect on women prone to hayfever and asthma triggered by flower pollen – psychosomatic effect Need to ensure essential oil is used, not the *absolute*, which is too concentrated for pregnancy use May be adulterated – purchase from reputable supplier (expensive)
Evidence base	Relaxing (Igarashi *et al.* 2014) Reduces anxiety in first-stage labour (Kheirkhah *et al.* 2014) Transdermal use relaxes and reduces stress (Hongratanaworakit 2009) Reduces fatigue (Varney and Buckle 2013) Reduces postnatal depression (Conrad and Adams 2012) May be useful for post-operative pain (Marofi *et al.* 2015) Reduces dysmenorrhoea (Sadeghi Aval Shahr *et al.* 2015)

Spearmint (*Mentha spicata*) – herb oil

Chemistry	l-carvone, limonene, β-myrcene, dihydrocarvone, 1.8 cineole, menthone, 3-octanol
Blends well with	Bergamot, chamomile, clary sage, cypress, eucalyptus, frankincense, geranium, grapefruit, jasmine, lavender, lime, mandarin/tangerine, neroli, orange (sweet), peppermint, rose, tea tree, ylang ylang Lovely fresh aroma, slightly sharper and lighter than peppermint – an excellent alternative for women who dislike peppermint but want the benefits of a mint oil
Reported effects	Similar to peppermint but limited documented evidence, even anecdotal Considered to be generally safer than peppermint
Indications	**Pregnancy** Nausea, vomiting, heartburn, indigestion, irritable bowel syndrome, constipation Muscular aches and pains, headaches Stress, anxiety Colds, influenza, sinus congestion Skin irritation **Labour** Pain relief Nausea, vomiting **Postnatal** Nausea, constipation, diarrhoea, flatulence, heartburn Recovery from birth Uplifting Tiredness, fatigue Pain relief
Contraindications and precautions	May cause skin irritation – maximum recommended dose 1.7% (Tisserand and Young 2014) Avoid in women with susceptibility to skin irritation Do not use with, or store next to, homeopathic remedies (inactivates them) It is reported by Tisserand and Young (2014) that some spearmint oils may contain up to 1% of pulegone (see Chapter 4) although they do not feel this is of concern, given the balance of other constituents which counteract any negative effects. However, it is wise to purchase from a reputable supplier and double-check that there is a minimal amount of pulegone in the oil.

Evidence base	Antibacterial – probably weak effect (Soković *et al.* 2010; Thompson *et al.* 2013) Anti-emetic (Hunt *et al.* 2013) May have anticonvulsive effect in epilepsy – animal research in early stages (Koutroumanidou *et al.* 2013)

Tea tree (*Melaleuca alternifolia*) – leaf oil

Chemistry	Terpinen-4-ol, α-terpineol, γ-terpinene, 1.8 cineole, pinene, α-terpenene, β-caryophyllene, ρ-cymene, aromadendrene, α-cadinene, limonene
Blends well with	Bergamot, chamomile, clary sage, cypress, eucalyptus, frankincense, geranium, grapefruit, jasmine, lavender lime, mandarin/tangerine, neroli, orange (sweet), peppermint, rose, spearmint, ylang ylang Strong, medical, camphorous, masculine aroma, which may need to be suppressed with other lighter and more fruity or floral aromas
Reported effects	Strongly antibacterial, antifungal, antiviral, antimicrobial, antiseptic Anti-inflammatory Antihypertensive Immunostimulant Decongestant
Indications	**Pregnancy** Leucorrhoea; vaginal thrush – low dilution in bath water Colds, influenza, bronchitis Acne, minor skin infections (e.g. verruca, spots, cold sores, abscess) Cystitis and urinary tract infection – suprapubic compress **Labour** DO NOT USE IN LABOUR **Postnatal** Perineal or abdominal wound infection Respiratory tract infection

Contraindications and precautions	*Do not use in labour* – thought to relax myometrium; may theoretically reduce contractions (Lis-Balchin 1999) Skin irritation possible with neat or prolonged dermal administration May cause mucus membrane irritation – avoid vaginal administration in pregnancy Oxidises rapidly if not stored well Avoid oral ingestion by children: may cause ataxia in high doses (Faiyazuddin *et al.* 2009) Do not use with or store next to homeopathic remedies (inactivates them)
Evidence base	Antibacterial (Dagli *et al.* 2015; Karbach *et al.* 2015) Antifungal (de Campos Rasteiro *et al.* 2014) Antibacterial, antiviral, antifungal, anti-inflammatory (Chin and Cordell 2013) Active against facial acne (Faiyazuddin *et al.* 2009) Effective against Candida albicans in conjunction with fluconazole (Di Vito *et al.* 2015; Mertas *et al.* 2015) Aids wound healing (Mertas *et al.* 2015) Active against MRSA (Edmondson *et al.* 2011; Warnke *et al.* 2013) Useful for facial acne (Hammer 2015; Pazyar *et al.* 2013) Antihypertensive Relaxes smooth muscle (Lis-Balchin *et al.* 1999) May cause contact dermatitis (Santesteban Muruzábal *et al.* 2015)

Ylang Ylang (*Cananga odorata*) – flower oil

Chemistry	Linalool, farnesol, geraniol, geranial, benzyl acetate, geranyl acetate, eugenol, methyl chavicol, methyl salicylate, pinene, β-caryophyllene, α-carophyllene, farnasene, δ-cadinene, benzyl benzoate
Blends well with	Bergamot, chamomile, clary sage, cypress, eucalyptus, frankincense, geranium, grapefruit, jasmine, lavender, lime, mandarin/tangerine, neroli, orange (sweet), peppermint, rose, spearmint, tea tree Deep aroma, which some find cloying but which is quite subtle; takes time to warm up and take effect; blends well with citrus, mint or floral aromas

Reported effects	Antidepressant, sedative, balancing, calming
	Aphrodisiac
	Antiseptic, antibacterial, antifungal
	Hypotensive
	Antispasmodic
	Reduces alertness
Indications	**Pregnancy**
	General wellbeing and relaxation
	Stress, fear, anxiety
	Insomnia, tiredness, fatigue, disturbed nights
	May help women with sexual dysfunction or relationship problems
	Mild to moderate hypotension
	Muscular cramps, gastrointestinal colic
	Prevention of infection
	Labour
	Pain relief – indirect effect may aid progress in labour
	Relaxation, anxiety, stress, fear, tension
	Postnatal
	General wellbeing and relaxation
	Prevention and treatment of 'blues', depression
	Aids recovery from birth and adaptation to parenthood
	Sexual and relationship problems, loss of libido
	Mild to moderate hypertension
	Prevention of infection
Contraindications and precautions	May be adulterated with cheaper oils — adulterated oil will become cloudy if put in refrigerator
	Avoid high doses and prolonged use – aroma may be overpowering
	Beware effect on women prone to hayfever and asthma triggered by flower pollen – psychosomatic effect
	Caution if postural/supine hypotension
	Caution with epidural anaesthesia
	Can have sedative effect or cause loss of concentration in staff
Evidence base	Reduces salivary cortisol and is harmonising – reduces blood pressure and heart rate, improves attention and alertness (Hongratanaworakit and Buchbauer 2004; Kim *et al.* 2012)
	Calming but decreases alertness, reaction time, memory and processing (Moss *et al.* 2006)
	Reduces concentration and memory due to relaxation (Moss *et al.* 2008)
	Transdermal absorption reduces blood pressure and increases skin temperature (Hongratanaworakit and Buchbauer 2006)
	Anti-infective (Tan *et al.* 2015)

Table 7.1 Principal therapeutic effects of essential oils (see also Chapter 3)

THERAPEUTIC EFFECT	NOTABLE ESSENTIAL OILS
Analgesic	Bergamot Black pepper (strong) Chamomile Frankincense (indirect) Lavender (moderate) Orange, sweet Peppermint Rose (mild)
Antibacterial NB All essential oils have some antibacterial action	Cypress Eucalyptus Lavender Tea tree
Anticoagulant (mild)	Bergamot Grapefruit Lime Mandarin/tangerine Neroli
Antidepressant	Bergamot Clary sage Frankincense Lavender (indirect) Ylang ylang (caution)
Anti-emetic	Bergamot Black pepper (caution, strong aroma) Grapefruit Lime Mandarin/tangerine Neroli Orange, sweet Peppermint Spearmint
Antifungal	Bergamot Eucalyptus Geranium Tea tree

cont.

THERAPEUTIC EFFECT	NOTABLE ESSENTIAL OILS
Antispasmodic	Bergamot Chamomile (strong) Clary sage Grapefruit Jasmine Lavender Lime Mandarin/tangerine Neroli Orange, sweet Peppermint Spearmint Ylang ylang
Antiviral **NB Evidence from *in vitro* research**	Bergamot Black pepper Eucalyptus Geranium
Astringent	Cypress Eucalyptus Lime Tea tree
Digestive aid	Bergamot Black pepper Chamomile Grapefruit Lime Mandarin/tangerine Neroli Orange, sweet Peppermint Spearmint
Expectorant	Black pepper Eucalyptus Frankincense Lavender Peppermint Spearmint Tea tree

Hypotensive	Bergamot Chamomile (indirect) Clary sage Frankincense (indirect) Lavender Ylang ylang
Laxative	Bergamot Black pepper Lavender Lime Mandarin/tangerine Neroli Orange, sweet Peppermint Spearmint
Relaxing	Bergamot Geranium Lavender Neroli Rose
Sedative (deeper effect than relaxing)	Chamomile Clary sage Frankincense Ylang ylang
Stimulating	Bergamot (circulation, digestive tract, mood) Black pepper (circulation) Cypress (vascular system) Eucalyptus (respiratory system) Geranium (psychological) Lime (circulation, digestive tract, mood) Mandarin/tangerine (digestive tract, mood) Peppermint (digestive tract, circulation) Spearmint (digestive tract, circulation) Tea tree (immune system)
Uterine relaxant (avoid in labour)	Tea tree
Uterine stimulant/ emmenagoguic (avoid until term)	Clary sage Lavender (mild) Jasmine Rose (mild)

Carrier oils

Essential oils are highly concentrated and, with only a few exceptions, should normally not be applied to the skin neat. This applies equally to using the essential oils in a massage blend or in water. The essential oils should be diluted in a good-quality vegetable oil, derived from plant or macerated herb oils. Mineral oils, such as baby oil, should not be used as they do not allow the essential oils to absorb into the skin adequately – they tend to sit on the surface of the skin and do not facilitate dispersion of the essential oils down the hair shafts. Some mineral oils may also contain lanolin, to which some people are allergic.

The carrier oil acts as a lubricant when performing massage to prevent the friction of skin-to-skin contact. There are many different carrier oils, which vary in texture, consistency and absorbency rates and are used for different purposes. All carrier oils have their own chemical constituents which give them therapeutic effects and add to the overall benefits of an aromatherapy treatment. They should be 100% pure and should not have too distinctive an aroma, which may overpower the aroma of the chosen therapeutic essential oils. Most carriers contain vitamins and minerals which help to nourish and moisturise the skin.

In maternity aromatherapy, it is not absolutely necessary to use a range of carrier oils unless the practitioner wishes to do so – for ease of practice a single carrier can be used. Grapeseed (*Vitis vinferi*) is one of the most universally acceptable and one of the most inexpensive carrier oils. It is obtained from the seeds of grapes, is yellow-green in colour, has a very light, non-greasy texture and no noticeable odour. Grapeseed oil has the correct consistency for massage and has the added advantage of washing out of towels and linen more easily than some of the other carriers.

Sweet almond oil (*Prunus amygdalis*) is derived from the kernels of sweet almonds and should not be confused with bitter almond oil – the latter may contain prussic acid or cyanide (hydrocyanic acid), which is produced during the extraction process. Sweet almond is usually greenish in colour but this may vary according to the time of harvesting (sometimes it can be a deep golden colour). Unrefined oil contains vitamins A, B1, B2, B6 and E, various minerals and mono- and polyunsaturated fats. If the oil is completely colourless, it is likely to have been refined and will no longer contain these nutrients. It is slightly sticky in texture and can be used on its own or combined with another carrier. However, care must be taken to ask each mother whether or not she has an allergy specifically to almonds, since sweet almond oil contains benzyl aldehyde, to which around 1% of the population is allergic.

Apricot kernel (*Prunus armeniaca*) and peach kernel (*Prunus persica*) carrier oils are produced from the seed kernels and are high in essential fatty acids, although unlike the fruit, they do not contain many vitamins, except vitamin E. Both oils, which are very pale in colour, are suitable for facial massage, for abdominal massage in pregnancy and labour and for dry, sensitive and mature skin. Apricot kernel oil may have an anti-inflammatory effect, making it a useful carrier for women with irritable bowel syndrome (Minaiyan *et al.* 2014).

Two carrier oils which are of a much thicker consistency and need to be diluted into a thinner oil such as grapeseed are avocado (*Persea americana*) and wheatgerm (*Triticum vulgare*). Unrefined avocado oil is deep green in colour and full of vitamins, lecithin, protein and essential fatty acids. It has a tendency to become cloudy and thick and, when cold, to solidify, leading producers in the cosmetics industry to refine it, after which it is no longer suitable for clinical aromatherapy. Wheatgerm oil is dark orange-brown in colour, thick, rich and very nourishing due to the vitamin E and essential fatty acids. The vitamin E also makes it a natural anti-oxidant, helping to prevent oxidation. Wheatgerm can be added to another carrier oil, in a ratio of approximately 1:4 to provide a nourishing carrier for dry skin. It will also prolong the 'shelf life' of an oil blend containing another carrier and several essential oils.

There are many other carrier oils available, but these are not essential to maternity aromatherapy. Coconut oil is also popular, but must be unrefined. It provides good lubrication, has a good effect in softening and moisturising the skin but leaves a slightly greasy film. As with essential oils, all carrier oils intended to be used for clinical aromatherapy should be purchased from a reputable supplier (not the local supermarket or market) and should be pure. Evening primrose oil is not normally used as a lubricant on its own but can be combined with another carrier in a ratio of 1:5. It is also useful for dry skin and for conditions such as eczema. It is thought to improve skin elasticity and accelerate healing. Hazelnut oil is a good lubricant, nourishes the skin, stimulates the circulation and has a slightly astringent effect. It is, however, probably best avoided in pregnancy, at least in women with a personal or family history of nut allergy, even though there is no evidence of neonatal allergy arising as a result of using it in pregnancy. Jojoba oil is also popular, providing good lubrication. It has a protective effect, is anti-inflammatory, can be used for a range of skin conditions and is suitable for use on both dry and oily skins. Safflower, sesame and sunflower oils are inexpensive although they can be slightly sticky in texture. Olive oil is not normally used in clinical aromatherapy as it is heavy and sticky with a noticeable odour. Other carriers include borage, camellia, macadamia nut, calendula, rosehip seed, St John's wort and wild carrot oils.

Glossary

7-dehydrocholesterol – steroid precursor of vitamin D

Abortifacient – capable of inducing spontaneous miscarriage

Analgesic – pain relieving

Antibacterial/fungal/viral – destroys/inhibits growth of bacteria, fungi, viruses

Anticoagulant – inhibits clotting of blood

Antipruritic – relieves skin itching

Astringent – causes contraction of tissues

Ataxia – loss of full control of body movements

Carminative – relieves flatulence

Cicatrisant – promotes formation of scar tissue

Cochrane reviews – systematic reviews of primary healthcare research studies, considered the highest standard in evidence-based healthcare

Cytochrome – haem compounds bonded to proteins that aid electron transfer in many metabolic processes, especially cellular respiration

Cytotoxicity – toxic to cells

Decongestant – relieves respiratory congestion

Diuretic – aids urination/micturition

Emmenagogue – capable of promoting menstruation-like vaginal bleeding

Epidermis – outer layer of cells overlying the dermis

Epigastric – pertaining to upper central abdomen

Epileptiform – convulsions similar to epilepsy

Erythrocytes – red blood cells

Expectorant – aids expulsion of mucus from respiratory tract

Febrifuge – reduces fever

Frenulotomy – Tongue tie division

Gynaecomastia – enlargement of breasts in men

Haematocrit – ratio of the volume of red blood cells to the total volume of blood

Hepatotoxic – toxic to the liver

Hypotensive – reduces blood pressure

Hypertensive – increases blood pressure

Integumentary system – skin

Intrapartum – during labour

Keratin – fibrous protein forming the main structural constituent of hair and nails

Keratohyaline granules – protein granular structure in the stratum granulosum of the epidermis, involved in keratinization

Laxative – promotes bowel movement

Lipophilic – able to combine with or dissolve in lipids or fats

Menorrhagia – excessively heavy menstruation

Moxibustion – Chinese medicine technique to turn breech–presenting fetus to head-first

Mutagenic – capable of causing mutations

Myometrium – muscle layer of uterus

Neurotoxic – toxic to nervous system

Pharmacokinetics – branch of pharmacology concerned with movement of drugs within the body

Photosensitivity – sensitive to ultraviolet sunlight

Photoxicity – capable of causing photosensitivity

Physiological hydraemia – increased fluid volume, with reduced concentration of red blood cells, giving rise to apparent anaemia with reduced haemoglobin levels; not normally a clinical problem

Reflexology – complementary therapy based on the concept of using one small part of the body as a 'micro-map' of the whole; applied pressure to specific points on the feet or hands relay stimuli to other parts of the body to treat various conditions

Rubefacient – increases local blood supply, causing reddening of the skin

Sedative – relaxing, promotes sleep

Stratified squamous epithelial tissue – epithelial cells arranged in layers upon a basal membrane. Only one layer is in contact with the basement membrane; the other layers adhere to one another to maintain structural integrity

Stratum basale – stratum basale (basal layer) is the deepest layer of the five epidermis layers, which is the outer covering of skin

Stratum corneum – outermost layer of the skin, consisting of keratinised cells

Stratum granulosum – thin layer of cells in the epidermis

Stratum lucidum – thin, clear layer of dead skin cells in the epidermis

Stratum spinosum – layer of epidermis of the skin between the stratum granulosum and stratum basale

Striae gravidarum – stretch marks

Teratogenic – agents capable of causing birth defects during development of the fetus

Volatile – substance capable of evaporating when exposed to air

Resources

Useful websites

www.a-t-c.org.uk Aromatherapy Trade Council – trade association for the essential oil trade, representing manufacturers and suppliers of aromatherapy products and the interests of consumers

www.cnhc.org.uk Complementary and Natural Healthcare Council – protects the public by providing UK voluntary register of complementary therapists; approved as an Accredited Register by the Professional Standards Authority for health and social care

www.expectancy.co.uk Expectancy – leading provider of courses on complementary therapies in pregnancy and childbirth, plus a range of professional and educational products

www.ifparoma.org/index.php International Federation of Professional Aromatherapists – one of the largest professional aromatherapy practitioner organisations in the world

www.nccam.nih.gov/research/camonpubmed Free database literature searching facility, focusing on complementary medicine research, but with access also to general healthcare research

Training courses

www.expectancy.co.uk/professional Courses in aromatherapy and massage for midwives, doulas, antenatal teachers and maternity nurses, and for aromatherapists and other complementary therapy practitioners wanting to work with pregnant women including:

- aromatherapy in midwifery practice three-day taught course, accredited by the Royal College of Midwives and the Federation of Antenatal Educators

- aromatherapy in maternity care four-day taught course for aromatherapists and massage therapists, accredited by the Federation of Holistic Therapists
- aromatherapy in midwifery practice two- or three-day taught course, available on your own premises, in the United Kingdom and overseas
- using essential oils in midwifery practice home study course
- aromatherapy workbook (home study) for continuing professional development.

Educational resources

www.expectancy.co.uk/shop A range of educational resources to aid the implementation and practice of aromatherapy when working with pregnant, labouring and newly birthed mothers, including:

- information leaflets for expectant mothers on the safe use of aromatherapy in pregnancy and birth, available as single downloads or on USB for unlimited download
- aromatherapy in midwifery e-book including profiles of 16 essential oils
- draft clinical guidelines (e-book or hard copy) to assist with the implementation of aromatherapy in midwifery practice, particularly within the NHS
- aromatherapy in maternity care poster for use in clinical practice
- aromatherapy in midwifery care guide to cascade training (e-leaflet)
- aromatherapy visitor awareness for use in birthing rooms (e-leaflet)
- professional starter pack for midwives and birth workers using aromatherapy in their practice
- client consultation forms for download
- door hangers stating 'Complementary therapies in progress, do not disturb'
- a range of educational products on other complementary therapies related to maternity care.

References

Abbaspoor Z and Mohammadkhani SL 2013 Lavender aromatherapy massages in reducing labor pain and duration of labor: A randomized controlled trial. *African Journal of Pharmacy and Pharmacology 7*(8): 426–30.

Abd Kadir SL, Yaakob H and Zulkifli MR 2013 Potential anti-dengue medicinal plants: A review. *J. Nat. Med. 67*(4): 677–89.

Adams J, Frawley J, Steel A, Broom A and Sibbritt D 2015 Use of pharmacological and non-pharmacological labour pain management techniques and their relationship to maternal and infant birth outcomes: Examination of a nationally representative sample of 1835 pregnant women. *Midwifery 31*(4): 458–63.

Adib-Hajbaghery M, Rajabi-Beheshtabad R and Abasi A 2013 Effect of whole body massage by patient's companion on the level of blood cortisol in coronary patients. *Nurs. Midwifery Stud. 2*(3): 10–15.

Adorjan B and Buchbauer G 2010 Biological properties of essential oils: An updated review. *Flavour and Fragrance Journal 25*: 407–26.

Agatonovic-Kustrin S, Babazadeh Ortakand D, Morton DW and Yusof AP 2015 Rapid evaluation and comparison of natural products and antioxidant activity in calendula, feverfew, and German chamomile extracts. *J. Chromatogr. A. 1385*: 103–10.

Aibinu I, Adenipekun T, Adelowotan T, Ogunsanya T and Odugbemi T 2006 Evaluation of the antimicrobial properties of different parts of Citrus aurantifolia (lime fruit) as used locally. *Afr. J. Tradit. Complement. Altern. Med. 4*(2): 185–90.

Al-Harrasi A, Ali L, Hussain J, Rehman NU, Mehjabeen, Ahmed M and Al-Rawahi A 2014 Analgesic effects of crude extracts and fractions of Omani frankincense obtained from traditional medicinal plant Boswellia sacra on animal models. *Asian Pac. J. Trop. Med. 7S1*: S485–90.

Alyssa Parian BN 2015 Dietary supplement therapies for inflammatory bowel disease: Crohn's disease and ulcerative colitis. *Curr. Pharm. Des. 22*(2): 180–8.

Amato A, Liotta R and Mulè F 2014 Effects of menthol on circular smooth muscle of human colon: Analysis of the mechanism of action. *Eur. J. Pharmacol. 740*: 295–301.

Andres C, Chen WC, Ollert M, Mempel M, Darsow U and Ring J 2009 Anaphylactic reaction to camomile tea. *Allergol. Int. 58*(1): 135–6.

Anzai A, Vázquez Herrera NE and Tosti A 2015 Airborne allergic contact dermatitis caused by chamomile tea. *Contact Dermatitis 72*(4): 254–5.

Arjouni MY, Bahri F, Romane A and El Fels MA 2011 Chemical composition and antimicrobial activity of essential oil of Cupressus atlantica. *Nat. Prod. Commun. 6*(10): 1519–22.

Asgary S, Naderi GA, Shams Ardekani MR, Sahebkar A *et al.* 2013 Chemical analysis and biological activities of Cupressus sempervirens var. horizontalis essential oils. *Pharm. Biol. 51*(2): 137–44.

Asnaashari S, Delazar A, Habibi B, Vasfi R *et al.* 2010 Essential oil from Citrus aurantifolia prevents ketotifen-induced weight-gain in mice. *Phytother. Res. 24*(12): 1893–7.

Ayan M, Tas U, Sogut E, Suren M, Gurbuzler L and Koyuncu F 2013 Investigating the effect of aromatherapy in patients with renal colic. *J. Altern. Complement. Med. 19*(4): 329–33.

Azanchi T, Shafaroodi H and Asgarpanah J 2014 Anticonvulsant activity of Citrus aurantium blossom essential oil (neroli): Involvment of the GABAergic system. *Nat. Prod. Commun. 9*(11): 1615–18.

Azimi H, Fallah-Tafti M, Karimi-Darmiyan M and Abdollahi M 2011 A comprehensive review of vaginitis phytotherapy. *Pak. J. Bio.l Sci. 14*(21): 960–6.

Babycentre 2011 Survey on the use of herbal medicines in pregnancy. Accessed at www. babycentre.co.uk/midwives/natural-remedies-survey, on 12 July 2011.

Bagetta G, Morrone LA, Rombolà L, Amantea D *et al.* 2010 Neuropharmacology of the essential oil of bergamot. *Fitoterapia 81*(6): 453–61.

Bagheri-Nesami M, Espahbodi F, Nikkhah A, Shorofi SA and Charati JY 2014 The effects of lavender aromatherapy on pain following needle insertion into a fistula in hemodialysis patients. *Complement. Ther. Clin. Pract. 20*(1): 1–4.

Bailey ML, Chudgar SM, Engle DL, Moon SD, Grochowski CO and Clay AS 2015 The impact of a mandatory immersion curriculum in integrative medicine for graduating medical students. *Explore (NY) 11*(5): 394–400.

Baird B, Murray R, Seale B, Foot C and Perry C 2015 *Midwifery Regulation in the United Kingdom.* London: The King's Fund.

Bakhtshirin F, Abedi S, YusefiZoj P and Razmjooee D 2015 The effect of aromatherapy massage with lavender oil on severity of primary dysmenorrhea in Arsanjan students. *Iran. J. Nurs. Midwifery Res. 20*(1): 156–60.

Bastard J and Tiran D 2006 Aromatherapy and massage for antenatal anxiety: Its effect on the fetus. *Complement. Ther. Clin. Pract. 12*(1): 48–54.

Bataller-Sifre R and Bataller-Alberola A 2015 What does integrative medicine provide to daily scientific clinical care? *Rev. Clin. Esp. 215*(8): 451–3.

Bayisa B, Tatiparthi R and Mulisa E 2014 Use of herbal medicine among pregnant women on antenatal care at Nekemte Hospital, Western Ethiopia. *Jundishapur J. Nat. Pharm. Prod. 9*(4): e1736.

BBC News 2009 Aromatherapy midwife struck off. Available at http://news.bbc.co.uk/1/ hi/wales/north_east/8189597.stm, accessed on 14 March 2016.

BBC News 2015 Homeopathy 'could be blacklisted'. Available at www.bbc.co.uk/news/ health-34744858, accessed on 14 March 2015.

Ben-Arye E, Schiff E, Raz OG, Samuels N and Lavie O 2014 Integrating a complementary medicine consultation for women undergoing chemotherapy. *Int. J. Gynaecol. Obstet. 124*(1): 51–4.

Ben Hassine D, Abderrabba M, Yvon Y, Lebrihi A *et al.* 2012 Chemical composition and in vitro evaluation of the antioxidant and antimicrobial activities of Eucalyptus gillii essential oil and extracts. *Molecules 17*(8): 9540–58.

Bercaw J, Maheshwari B and Sangi-Haghpeykar H 2010 The use during pregnancy of prescription, over-the-counter, and alternative medications among Hispanic women. *Birth* 37(3): 211–18.

Bikmoradi A, Seifi Z, Poorolajal J, Araghchian M, Safiaryan R and Oshvandi K 2015 Effect of inhalation aromatherapy with lavender essential oil on stress and vital signs in patients undergoing coronary artery bypass surgery: A single-blinded randomized clinical trial. *Complement. Ther. Med.* 23(3): 331–8.

Birdee GS, Kemper KJ, Rothman R and Gardiner P 2014 Use of complementary and alternative medicine during pregnancy and the postpartum period: An analysis of the National Health Interview Survey. *J. Women's Health (Larchmt)* 23(10): 824–9.

Birth Choice UK 2014. Available at www.birthchoiceuk.com/Professionals/index.html, accessed on 14 March 2016.

Bishop JL, Northstone K, Green JR and Thompson EA 2011 The use of complementary and alternative medicine in pregnancy: Data from the Avon longitudinal study of parents and children (ALSPAC). *Complement. Ther. Med.* 19(6): 303–10.

Blumenthal M, Goldberg A and Brinckman J (eds) 2000 *Herbal Medicine: Expanded Commission E Monographs*. Austin, TX: American Botanical Council.

Boitor M, Martorella G, Arbour C, Michaud C and Gélinas C 2015 Evaluation of the preliminary effectiveness of hand massage therapy on postoperative pain of adults in the intensive care unit after cardiac surgery: A pilot randomized controlled trial. *Pain Manag, Nurs.* 16(3): 354–66.

Bond S 2014 Pregnant women use non-professional sources when seeking information about complementary and alternative practices. *J. Midwifery Women's Health* 59(6): 669.

Boukhatem MN, Ferhat MA, Kameli A, Saidi F and Kebir HT 2014 Lemon grass (Cymbopogon citratus) essential oil as a potent anti-inflammatory and antifungal drugs. Libyan J. Med. doi: 10.3402/ljm.v9.25431.

Boukhatem MN, Kameli A, Ferhat MA, Saidi F and Mekarnia M 2013 Rose geranium essential oil as a source of new and safe anti-inflammatory drugs. *Libyan J. Med.* 8: 22520.

Boukhris M, Bouaziz M, Feki I, Jemai H, El Feki A and Sayadi S 2012 Hypoglycemic and antioxidant effects of leaf essential oil of Pelargonium graveolens L'Hér. in alloxan induced diabetic rats. *Lipids Health Dis.* 11: 81.

Buchbauer G 1996 Methods in aromatherapy research. *Perfumer and Flavorist* 21: 31–6.

Burns E, Zobbi V, Panzeri D, Oskrochi R and Regalia A 2007 Aromatherapy in childbirth: A pilot randomised controlled trial. *BJOG* 114(7): 838–44.

Burns EE, Blamey C, Ersser SJ, Barnetson L and Lloyd AJ 2000 An investigation into the use of aromatherapy in intrapartum midwifery practice. *J. Altern. Complement. Med.* 6(2): 141–7.

Butt MS, Pasha I, Sultan MT, Randhawa MA, Saeed F and Ahmed W 2013 Black pepper and health claims: A comprehensive treatise. *Crit. Rev. Food Sci. Nutr.* 53(9): 875–86.

Caldeira S, Timmins F, de Carvalho EC and Vieira M 2015 Nursing diagnosis of 'spiritual distress' in women with breast cancer: Prevalence and major defining characteristics. *Cancer Nurs.* Oct 22.

Cappello G, Spezzaferro M, Gross I, Manzoli L and Marzio L 2007 Peppermint oil (Mintoil) in the treatment of irritable bowel syndrome: A prospective, double-blind, placebo-controlled randomised trial. *Dig. Liv. Dis.* 39: 530–6.

Carmen G and Hancu G 2014 Antimicrobial and antifungal activity of pelargonium roseum essential oils. *Adv. Pharm. Bull.* 4(2): 511–14.

Cash BD, Epstein MS and Shah SM 2015 A novel delivery system of peppermint oil is an effective therapy for irritable bowel syndrome symptoms. *Dig. Dis. Sci.* 61(2): 560–71.

Chandwani KD, Heckler CE, Mohile SG, Mustian KM *et al.* 2014 Hot flashes severity, complementary and alternative medicine use, and self-rated health in women with breast cancer. *Explore (NY)* 10(4): 241–7.

Chang KM and Shen CW 2011 Aromatherapy benefits autonomic nervous system regulation for elementary school faculty in Taiwan. *Evid. Based Complement. Alternat. Med.* doi: 10.1155/2011/946537.

Chang SM and Chen CH 2015 Effects of an intervention with drinking chamomile tea on sleep quality and depression in sleep disturbed postnatal women: A randomized controlled trial. *J. Adv. Nurs.* Oct 20.

Chen FP, Chang CM, Shiu JH, Chiu JH, Wu TP, Yang J *et al.* 2015 A clinical study of integrating acupuncture and Western medicine in treating patients with Parkinson's disease. *Am. J. Chin. Med.* 43(3): 407–23.

Chen SL and Chen CH 2015 Effects of lavender tea on fatigue, depression, and maternal-infant attachment in sleep-disturbed postnatal women. Worldviews *Evid. Based Nurs.* 12(6): 370–9.

Chen MC, Fang SH and Fang L 2015 The effects of aromatherapy in relieving symptoms related to job stress among nurses. *Int. J. Nurs. Pract.* 21(1): 87–93.

Chin KB and Cordell B 2013 The effect of tea tree oil (Melaleuca alternifolia) on wound healing using a dressing model. *J. Altern Complement Med.* 19(12): 942–5.

Chioca LR, Antunes VD, Ferro MM, Losso EM and Andreatini R 2013 Anosmia does not impair the anxiolytic-like effect of lavender essential oil inhalation in mice. *Life Sci.* 92(20–21): 971–5.

Choi SY, Kang P, Lee HS and Seol GH 2014 Effects of inhalation of essential oil of citrus aurantium l. var. amara on menopausal symptoms, stress, and estrogen in postmenopausal women: A randomized controlled trial. *Evid. Based Complement. Alternat. Med.* doi: 10.1155/2014/796518.

Conrad P and Adams C 2012 The effects of clinical aromatherapy for anxiety and depression in the high risk postpartum woman – a pilot study. *Complement. Ther. Clin. Pract.* 18(3): 164–8.

Constant D, Grossman D, Lince N and Harries J 2014 Self-induction of abortion among women accessing second-trimester abortion services in the public sector, Western Cape Province, South Africa: An exploratory study. *S. Afr. Med. J.* 104(4): 302–5.

Corazza M, Borghi A, Gallo R, Schena D *et al.* 2014 Topical botanically derived products: Use, skin reactions, and usefulness of patch tests: A multicentre Italian study. *Contact Dermatitis* 70(2): 90–7.

Cordell B and Buckle J 2013 The effects of aromatherapy on nicotine craving on a US campus: A small comparison study. *J. Altern. Complement. Med.* 19(8): 709–13.

Cosentino M, Luini A, Bombelli R, Corasaniti MT, Bagetta G and Marino F 2014 The essential oil of bergamot stimulates reactive oxygen species production in human polymorphonuclear leukocytes. *Phytother. Res.* 28(8): 1232–9.

Coyle ME, Smith CA and Peat B 2012 Cephalic version by moxibustion for breech presentation. *Cochrane Database Syst. Rev.* doi: 10.1002/14651858.CD003928.pub3.

Cragan JD, Friedman JM, Holmes LB, Uhi K, Green NS and Riley L 2006 Ensuring the safe and effective use of medications during pregnancy: Planning and prevention through preconception care. *Maternal and Child Health* 10(5): S129–35.

Crandon KL and Thompson JP 2006 Olbas oil and respiratory arrest in a child. *Clinical Toxicology* 44: 568.

Crane JD, Ogborn DI, Cupido C, Melov S *et al.* 2012 Massage therapy attenuates inflammatory signaling after exercise-induced muscle damage. *Sci. Transl. Med.* 4(119): 119ra13.

Crawford GH, Katz KA, Ellis E and James WD 2004 Use of aromatherapy products and increased risk of hand dermatitis in massage therapists *Arch. Dermatol.* 140: 991–6.

Crowther S 2013 Sacred space at the moment of birth. *Pract. Midwife* 16(11): 21–3.

Cullen JG 2015 Nursing management, religion and spirituality: A bibliometric review, a research agenda and implications for practice. *J. Nurs. Manag.* 24(3): 291–9.

Dagli N, Dagli R, Mahmoud RS and Baroudi K 2015 Essential oils, their therapeutic properties, and implication in dentistry: A review. *J. Int. Soc. Prev. Community Dent.* 5(5): 335–40.

Dahlen HG, Tracy S, Tracy M, Bisits A, Brown C and Thornton C 2012 Rates of obstetric intervention among low-risk women giving birth in private and public hospitals in NSW: A population-based descriptive study. *BMJ Open* doi: 10.1136/bmjopen-2013-004551.

Davies SJ, Harding LM and Baranowski AP 2002 A novel treatment of postherpetic neuralgia using peppermint oil. *Clin. J. Pain*18(3): 200–2.

Davies P 1991 *Subtle Aromatherapy*. Saffron Walden: CW Daniel.

de Campos Rasteiro VM, da Costa AC, Araújo CF, de Barros PP *et al.* 2014 Essential oil of Melaleuca alternifolia for the treatment of oral candidiasis induced in an immunosuppressed mouse model. *BMC Complement. Altern. Med.* 14: 489. Available at www.ncbi.nlm.nih.gov/pmc/articles/PMC4301879, accessed on 7 May 2016.

de Sousa DP, Hocayen P de A, Andrade LN and Andreatini R 2015 A systematic review of the anxiolytic-like effects of essential oils in animal models. *Molecules* 20(10): 18620–60.

De Vincenzi M, De Vincenzi A and Silano M 2004 Constituents of aromatic plants: Elemicin. *Fitoterapia* 75(6): 615–18.

Dhany AL, Mitchell T and Foy C 2012 Aromatherapy and massage intrapartum service impact on use of analgesia and anesthesia in women in labor: A retrospective case note analysis. *J. Altern. Complement. Med.* 18(10): 932–8.

Dharmadhikari NP, Rao AR, Pimplikar SS, Kharat AG *et al.* 2010 Effect of geopathic stress on human heart rate and blood pressure. *Indian Journal of Science and Technology.* doi: 10.17485/ijst/2010/v3i1/29644.

Dias BG and Ressler KJ 2014 Parental olfactory experience influences behavior and neural structure in subsequent generations. *Nat Neurosci.* 17(1): 89–96.

Diaz A, Luque L, Badar Z, Kornic S and Danon M 2015 Prepubertal gynecomastia and chronic lavender exposure: Report of three cases. *J. Pediatr. Endocrinol. Metab. 29* (1):103–7.

Dick-Read G 2013 Childbirth without fear (2nd edn). London: Pinter and Martin.

Diego MA, Field T and Hernandez-Reif M 2014 Preterm infant weight gain is increased by massage therapy and exercise via different underlying mechanisms. *Early Hum. Dev. 90*(3): 137–40.

Di Vito M, Mattarelli P, Modesto M, Girolamo A *et al.* F 2015 In vitro activity of tea tree oil vaginal suppositories against Candida spp. and probiotic vaginal microbiota. *Phytother. Res. 29*(10): 1628–33.

Domaracký M, Rehák P, Juhás S and Koppel J 2007 Effects of selected plant essential oils on the growth and development of mouse pre-implantation embryos in vivo. *Physiol. Res. 56*(1): 97–104.

Downe 2014 Better births and the physiological processes for labour and birth Available at www.rcm.org.uk/why-normal-births-and-normalisation-of-the-process-is-so-important, accessed on 14 March 2016.

Ebihara T, Ebihara S, Maruyama M, Kobayashi M *et al.* 2006 A randomized trial of olfactory stimulation using black pepper oil in older people with swallowing dysfunction. *J. Am. Geriatr. Soc. 54*(9): 1401–6.

Edmondson M, Newall N, Carville K, Smith J, Riley TV and Carson CF 2011 Uncontrolled, open-label, pilot study of tea tree (Melaleuca alternifolia) oil solution in the decolonisation of methicillin-resistant Staphylococcus aureus positive wounds and its influence on wound healing. *Int. Wound J. 8*(4): 375–84.

Elaissi A, Rouis Z, Salem NA, Mabrouk S *et al.* 2012 Chemical composition of eight eucalyptus species' essential oils and the evaluation of their antibacterial, antifungal and antiviral activities. *BMC Complement. Altern. Med. 12*: 81.

Esposito ER, Bystrek MV and Klein JS 2014 An elective course in aromatherapy science. *Am. J. Pharm. Educ. 78*(4): 79.

Faiyazuddin MD, Suri S, Mustafa G, Iqbal Z *et al.* 2009 Phytotherapeutic potential of tea tree essential oil in vitro and energising vistas in the skincare industry: A comprehensive review. *International Journal of Essential Oil Therapeutics 3*(2–3): 84–90.

Falk-Filipsson A, Löf A, Hagberg M, Hjelm EW and Wang Z 1993 δ-limonene exposure to humans by inhalation: Uptake, distribution, elimination and effects on the pulmonary system. *Journal of Toxicology and Environmental Health 38*: 77–8.

Faturi CB, Leite JR, Alves PB, Canton AC and Teixeira-Silva F 2010 Anxiolytic-like effect of sweet orange aroma in Wistar rats. *Prog. Neuropsychopharmacol. Biol. Psychiatry 34*(4): 605–9.

Feijen-de Jong EI, Jansen DE, Baarveld F, Spelten E, Schellevis F and Reijneveld SA 2015 Determinants of use of care provided by complementary and alternative health care practitioners to pregnant women in primary midwifery care: A prospective cohort study. *BMC Pregnancy Childbirth 15*: 140.

Fernández LF, Palomino OM and Frutos G 2014 Effectiveness of Rosmarinus officinalis essential oil as anti-hypotensive agent in primary hypotensive patients and its influence on health-related quality of life. *J. Ethnopharmacol. 151*(1): 509–16.

Field T 2014 Massage therapy research review. *Complement. Ther. Clin. Pract.* 20(4): 224–9.

Field T, Diego M and Hernandez-Reif M 2010 Moderate pressure is essential for massage therapy effects. *Int J Neurosci.* *120*(5): 381–5.

Field T, Diego M, Hernandez-Reif M, Deeds O and Figueiredo B 2009 Pregnancy massage reduces prematurity, low birthweight and postpartum depression. *Infant Behav. Dev.* *32*(4): 454–60.

Field T, Diego MA, Hernandez-Reif M, Schanberg S and Kuhn C 2004 Massage therapy effects on depressed pregnant women. *J. Psychosom. Obstet. Gynaecol.* *25*(2): 115–22.

Field T, Hernandez-Reif M, Diego M, Schanberg S and Kuhn C 2005 Cortisol decreases and serotonin and dopamine increase following massage therapy. *Int. J. Neurosci.* *115*(10): 1397–413.

Finny P, Stephen C, Jacob R, Tharyan P and Seshadri MS 2015 Jasmine flower extract lowers prolactin. *Tropical Doctor* *45*(2): 118–22.

Flaherty G, Fitzgibbon J and Cantillon P 2015 Attitudes of medical students toward the practice and teaching of integrative medicine. *J. Integr. Med.* *13*(6): 412–15.

Foster E 2006 The spiritual encounter within a complementary therapy treatment. *Complement. Ther. Clin. Pract.* *12*(2): 163–9.

Frawley J, Adams J, Broom A, Steel A, Gallois C and Sibbritt D 2014 Majority of women are influenced by nonprofessional information sources when deciding to consult a complementary and alternative medicine practitioner during pregnancy. *J. Altern. Complement. Med.* *20*(7): 571–7.

Frawley J, Adams J, Steel A, Broom A, Gallois C and Sibbritt D 2015 Women's use and self-prescription of herbal medicine during pregnancy: An examination of 1835 pregnant women. *Women's Health Issues* *25*(4): 396-402.

Fujita M, Endoh Y, Saimon N and Yamaguchi S 2006 Effect of massaging babies on mothers: Pilot study on the changes in mood states and salivary cortisol level. *Complement. Ther. Clin. Pract.* *12*(3): 181–5.

Gay CW, Robinson ME, George SZ, Perlstein WM and Bishop MD 2014 Immediate changes after manual therapy in resting-state functional connectivity as measured by functional magnetic resonance imaging in participants with induced low back pain. *J. Manipulative Physiol. Ther.* *37*(9): 614–27.

Goes TC, Antunes FD, Alves PB and Teixeira-Silva F 2012 Effect of sweet orange aroma on experimental anxiety in humans. *J. Altern. Complement. Med.* *18*(8): 798–804.

Greenway FL, Frome BM, Engels TM and MacLellan A 2003 Temporary relief of post-herpetic neuralgia pain with topical geranium oil. *American Journal of Medicine* *115*(7): 586–7.

Guimarães AG, Quintans JS and Quintans LJ Jr 2013 Monoterpenes with analgesic activity – a systematic review. *Phytother. Res.* *27*(1): 1–15.

Gyldenløve M, Menné T and Thyssen JP 2014 Eucalyptus contact allergy. *Contact Dermatitis* *71*(5): 303–4.

Hadi N and Hanid AA 2011 Lavender essence for post-cesarean pain. *Pak. J. Biol. Sci.* *14*(11): 664–7.

Hajibagheri A, Babaii A and Adib-Hajbaghery M 2014 Effect of Rosa damascene aromatherapy on sleep quality in cardiac patients: A randomized controlled trial. *Complement. Ther. Clin. Pract.* *20*(3): 159–63.

Hall HG, Griffiths DL and McKenna LG 2011 The use of complementary and alternative medicine by pregnant women: A literature review. *Midwifery* *27*(6): 817–24.

Hall HG, Griffiths DL and McKenna LG. 2012a Complementary and alternative medicine in midwifery practice: Managing the conflicts. *Complement. Ther. Clin. Pract.* *18*(4): 246–51.

Hall HG, Griffiths DL and McKenna LG 2013a Keeping childbearing safe: Midwives' influence on women's use of complementary and alternative medicine. *Int. J. Nurs. Pract.* *19*(4): 437–43.

Hall HG, Griffiths DL and McKenna LG 2013b Navigating a safe path together: A theory of midwives' responses to the use of complementary and alternative medicine. *Midwifery 29*(7): 801–8.

Hall HG, McKenna LG and Griffiths DL 2012b Midwives' support for complementary and alternative medicine: A literature review. *Women Birth 25*(1): 4–12.

Hammer KA 2015 Treatment of acne with tea tree oil (melaleuca) products: A review of efficacy, tolerability and potential modes of action. *Int. J. Antimicrob. Agents 45*(2): 106–10.

Haze S, Sakai K, Gozu Y and Moriyama M 2010 Grapefruit oil attenuates adipogenesis in cultured subcutaneous adipocytes. *Planta Med. 76*(10): 950–5.

Heidari Gorji MA, Ashrastaghi OG, Habibi V, Charati JY, Ebrahimzadeh MA and Ayasi M 2015 The effectiveness of lavender essence on sternotomy related pain intensity after coronary artery bypass grafting. *Adv. Biomed. Res. 4*: 127.

Henley DV, Lipson N, Korach KS and Bloch CA 2007 Prepubertal gynecomastia linked to lavender and tea tree oils. *N. Engl. J. Med. 356*(5): 479–85.

Herman A, Tambor K and Herman A 2015 Linalool affects the antimicrobial efficacy of essential oils. *Curr Microbiol. 72*(2): 165–72.

Herro E and Jacob SE 2010 Mentha piperita (peppermint). *Dermatitis 21*(6): 327–9.

Heuberger E, Hongratanaworakit T, Böhm C, Weber R and Buchbauer G 2001 Effects of chiral fragrances on human autonomic nervous system parameters and self-evaluation. *Chemical Senses 26*: 281–92.

Heuberger E and Ilmberger J 2010 The influence of essential oils on human vigilance. *Nat. Prod. Commun. 5*(9): 1441–6.

Hirsch AR, Ye Y, Lu Y and Choe M 2007b The effects of the aroma of jasmine on bowling score. *International Journal of Essential Oil Therapeutics 1*: 79–82.

Holden SC, Gardiner P, Birdee G, Davis RB and Yeh GY 2015 Complementary and alternative medicine use among women during pregnancy and childbearing years. *Birth* June 25.

Hongratanaworakit T 2009 The relaxing effect of rose oil on humans. *Nat. Prod. Commun. 4*(2): 291–6.

Hongratanaworakit T 2010 Stimulating effect of aromatherapy massage with jasmine oil. *Nat. Prod. Commun. 5*(1): 157–62.

Hongratanaworakit T 2011 Aroma-therapeutic effects of massage blended essential oils on humans. *Nat. Prod. Commun. 6*(8): 1199–204.

Hongratanaworakit T and Buchbauer G 2004 Evaluation of the harmonising effect of yanh ylang oil on humans after inhalation. *Planta Med. 70*: 632–6.

Hongratanaworakit T and Buchbauer G 2006 Relaxing effect of ylang ylang oil on humans after transdermal absorption. *Phytother. Res. 20*(9): 758–63.

House of Lords Select Committee on Science and Technology 2000 *Sixth Report on Complementary and Alternative Medicine*. London: HMSO.

Hunt KJ, Coelho HF, Wider B, Perry R *et al.* 2010 Complementary and alternative medicine use in England: Results from a national survey. *Int. J. Clin. Pract.* 64(11): 1496–502.

Hunt R, Dienemann J, Norton HJ, Hartley W *et al.* 2013 Aromatherapy as treatment for postoperative nausea: A randomized trial. *Anesth. Analg.* 117(3): 597–604.

Hwang E and Shin S 2015 The effects of aromatherapy on sleep improvement: A systematic literature review and meta-analysis. *J. Altern. Complement. Med.* 21(2): 61–8.

Igarashi M, Ikei H, Song C and Miyazaki Y 2014 Effects of olfactory stimulation with rose and orange oil on prefrontal cortex activity. *Complement. Ther. Med.* 22(6): 1027–31.

Ikeda H, Takasu S and Murase K 2014 Contribution of anterior cingulate cortex and descending pain inhibitory system to analgesic effect of lemon odor in mice. *Mol. Pain 10*: 14. doi: 10.1186/1744-8069-10-14.

Imura M, Misao H and Ushijima H 2006 The psychological effects of aromatherapy-massage in healthy postpartum mothers. *J. Midwifery Women's Health 51*(2): e21–7.

Ireland DJ, Greay SJ, Hooper CM, Kissick HT *et al.* 2012 Topically applied Melaleuca alternifolia (tea tree) oil causes direct anti-cancer cytotoxicity in subcutaneous tumour bearing mice. *J. Dermatol. Sci.* 67(2): 120–9.

Irmak Sapmaz H, Uysal M, Taş U, Esen M *et al.* S 2015 The effect of lavender oil in patients with renal colic: A prospective controlled study using objective and subjective outcome measurements. *J Altern Complement Med.* 21(10): 617–22.

Jacquemyn Y *et al.* 2012 Elective induction of labour increases caesarean section rate in low risk multiparous women. *J. Obstet. Gynaecol.* 32(3): 257–9.

Jafarzadeh M, Arman S and Pour FF 2013 Effect of aromatherapy with orange essential oil on salivary cortisol and pulse rate in children during dental treatment: A randomized controlled clinical trial. *Adv. Biomed. Res.* 2: 10. doi: 10.4103/2277-9175.107968.

Jain N and Astin JA 2001 Barriers to acceptance: An exploratory study of complementary/alternative disuse. *J. Altern. Complement. Med.* 7(6): 689–96.

Jamalian A, Shams-Ghahfarokhi M, Jaimand K, Pashootan N, Amani A and Razzaghi-Abyaneh M 2012 Chemical composition and antifungal activity of Matricaria recutita flower essential oil against medically important dermatophytes and soil-borne pathogens. *J Mycol Med.* 22(4): 308–15.

Janssen P, Shroff F and Jaspar P 2012 Massage therapy and labor outcomes: A randomized controlled trial. *Int. J. Ther. Massage Bodywork 5*(4): 15–20.

Jones L, Othman M, Dowswell T, Alfirevic Z *et al.* 2012 Pain management for women in labour: An overview of systematic reviews. *Cochrane Database Syst. Rev. 3*: CD009234.

Karadag E, Samancioglu S, Ozden D and Bakir E 2015 Effects of aromatherapy on sleep quality and anxiety of patients. *Nurs. Crit. Care.* doi: 10.1111/nicc.12198.

Karbach J, Ebenezer S, Warnke PH, Behrens E and Al-Nawas B 2015 Antimicrobial effect of Australian antibacterial essential oils as alternative to common antiseptic solutions against clinically relevant oral pathogens. *Clin. Lab.* 61(1–2): 61–8.

Kaviani M, Maghbool S, Azima S and Tabaei MH 2014 Comparison of the effect of aromatherapy with Jasminum officinale and Salvia officinale on pain severity and labor outcome in nulliparous women. *Iran. J. Nurs. Midwifery Res.* 19(6): 666–72.

Kearns GL, Chumpitazi BP, Abdel-Rahman SM, Garg U and Shulman RJ 2015 Systemic exposure to menthol following administration of peppermint oil to paediatric patients. *BMJ Open 5*(8): e008375.

Kehrl W, Sommermann U and Dethlefsen U 2004 Therapy for acute non-purulent rhinosinusitis with cineole: Results of a double-blind, randomised, placebo-controlled trial. *Laryngoscope 114*: 738–42.

Kennedy DA, Lupattelli A, Koren G and Nordeng H 2013 Herbal medicine use in pregnancy: Results of a multinational study. *BMC Complement Altern Med.* doi: 10.1186/1472-6882-13-355.

Keshavarz Afshar M, Behboodi Moghadam Z, Taghizadeh Z, Bekhradi R, Montazeri A and Mokhtari P 2015 Lavender fragrance essential oil and the quality of sleep in postpartum women. *Iran. Red Crescent Med. J. 17*(4): e25880.

Kheirkhah M, Vali Pour NS, Nisani L and Haghani H 2014 Comparing the effects of aromatherapy with rose oils and warm foot bath on anxiety in the first stage of labor in nulliparous women. *Iran. Red Crescent Med. J. 16*(9): e14455.

Khodabakhsh P, Shafaroodi H and Asgarpanah J 2015 Analgesic and anti-inflammatory activities of Citrus aurantium L. blossoms essential oil (neroli): Involvement of the nitric oxide/cyclic-guanosine monophosphate pathway. *J. Nat. Med. 69*(3): 324–31.

Kim IH, Kim C, Seong K, Hur MH, Lim HM and Lee MS 2012 Essential oil inhalation on blood pressure and salivary cortisol levels in pre-hypertensive and hypertensive subjects. *Evid. Based Complement. Alternat. Med.* doi: 10.1155/2012/984203.

Kim JT, Ren CJ, Fielding GA, Pitti A *et al.* 2007 Treatment with lavender aromatherapy in the post-anesthesia care unit reduces opioid requirements of morbidly obese patients undergoing laparoscopic adjustable gastric banding. *Obes. Surg. 17*(7): 920–5.

Kim JT, Wajda M, Cuff G, Serota D *et al.* 2006 Evaluation of aromatherapy in treating postoperative pain: Pilot study. *Pain Pract. 6*(4): 273–7.

King's Fund 2009 Safer birth: Everybody's business. An independent inquiry into the safety of maternity services in England. Available at www.kingsfund.org.uk/sites/files/kf/field/field_publication_file/safe-births-everybodys-business-onora-oneill-february-2008.pdf, accessed on 7 May 2016.

Kitikannakorn N, Chaiyakunapruk N, Nimpitakpong P, Dilokthornsakul P, Meepoo E and Kerdpeng W 2013 An overview of the evidences of herbals for smoking cessation. *Complement. Ther. Med. 21*(5): 557–64.

Kollndorfer K, Kowalczyk K, Nell S, Krajnik J, Mueller CA and Schöpf V 2015 The inability to self-evaluate smell performance. How the vividness of mental images outweighs awareness of olfactory performance. *Front Psychol.* doi: 10.3389/fpsyg.2015.00627.

Köteles F and Babulka P 2014 Role of expectations and pleasantness of essential oils in their acute effects. *Acta Physiol. Hung. 101*(3): 329–40.

Koutroumanidou E, Kimbaris A, Kortsaris A, Bezirtzoglou E *et al.* 2013 Increased seizure latency and decreased severity of pentylenetetrazol-induced seizures in mice after essential oil administration. *Epilepsy Res. Treat.* doi: 10.1155/2013/532657.

Kristiniak S, Harpel J, Breckenridge DM and Buckle J 2012 Black pepper essential oil to enhance intravenous catheter insertion in patients with poor vein visibility: A controlled study. *J. Altern. Complement. Med. 18*(11): 1003–7.

Kuroda K, Inoue N, Ito Y, Kubota K *et al.* 2005 Sedative effects of the jasmine tea odor and (R)-(-)-linalool, one of its major odor components, on autonomic nerve activity and mood states. *Eur. J. Appl. Physiol.* 95(2–3): 107–14.

Lavabre M 1990 *Aromatherapy Workbook.* Vermont: Healing Arts Press.

Laird K and Phillips C 2012 Vapour phase: A potential future use for essential oils as antimicrobials? *Lett. Appl. Microbiol.* 54(3): 169–74.

Lane B, Cannella K, Bowen C, Copelan D *et al.* 2012 Examination of the effectiveness of peppermint aromatherapy on nausea in women post C-section. *J. Holist. Nurs.* 30(2): 90–104.

Langhorst J, Wulfert H, Lauche R, Klose P *et al.* 2015 Systematic review of complementary and alternative medicine treatments in inflammatory bowel diseases. *J. Crohns Colitis* 9(1): 86–106.

Larson D and Jacob SE 2012 Tea tree oil. *Dermatitis* 23(1): 48–9.

Lee K, Lee JH, Kim SI, Cho MH and Lee J 2014a Anti-biofilm, anti-hemolysis, and anti-virulence activities of black pepper, cananga, myrrh oils, and nerolidol against Staphylococcus aureus. *Appl. Microbiol. Biotechnol.* 98(22): 9447–57.

Lee KB, Cho E and Kang YS 2014b Changes in 5-hydroxytryptamine and cortisol plasma levels in menopausal women after inhalation of clary sage oil. *Phytother. Res.* 28(11): 1599–605.

Lehrner J, Marwinski G, Lehr S, Johren P and Deecke L 2005 Ambient odors of orange and lavender reduce anxiety and improve mood in a dental office. *Physiol. Behav.* 86(1–2): 92–5.

Liao IC, Chen SL, Wang MY and Tsai PS 2014 Effects of massage on blood pressure in patients with hypertension and prehypertension: A meta-analysis of randomized controlled trials. *J. Cardiovasc. Nurs.* 31(1): 73–83.

Liddle SD and Pennick V 2015 Interventions for preventing and treating low-back and pelvic pain during pregnancy. *Cochrane Database Syst. Rev.* doi: 10.1002/14651858. CD001139.pub4.

Lillehei AS and Halcon LL 2014 A systematic review of the effect of inhaled essential oils on sleep. *J. Altern. Complement. Med.* 20(6): 441–51.

Lis-Balchin M 1999 Possible health and safety problems in the use of novel plant essential oils and extracts in aromatherapy. *J. R. Soc. Promot. Health* 119(4): 240–3.

Lis-Balchin M 2010 Aromatherapy and Essential Oils. In Hüsnü Can Baser and Buchbauer (eds) *Handbook of Essential Oils: Science, Technology and Applications.* Florida: CRC Press.

Lis-Balchin M, Hart SL and Deans SG 2000 Pharmacological and antimicrobial studies on different tea-tree oils (Melaleuca alternifolia, Leptospermum scoparium or Manuka and Kunzea ericoides or Kanuka), originating in Australia and New Zealand. *Phytother. Res.* 14(8): 623–9.

Lis-Balchin M, Hart S and Wan Hang Lo B 2002 Jasmine absolute (Jasminum grandiflora L.) and its mode of action on guinea-pig ileum in vitro. *Phytother. Res.* 16(5): 437–9.

Liu SH, Lin TH and Chang KM 2013 The physical effects of aromatherapy in alleviating work-related stress on elementary school teachers in Taiwan. *Evid. Based Complement. Alternat. Med.* doi: 10.1155/2013/853809.

Lua PL and Zakaria NS 2012 A brief review of current scientific evidence involving aromatherapy use for nausea and vomiting. *J. Altern. Complement. Med.* 18(6): 534–40.

Lytle J, Mwatha C and Davis KK 2014 Effect of lavender aromatherapy on vital signs and perceived quality of sleep in the intermediate care unit: A pilot study. *Am. J. Crit. Care 23*(1): 24–9.

Maddocks-Jennings W 2004 Critical incident: Idiosyncratic allergic reactions to essential oils. *Complement. Ther. Nurs. Midwifery 10*(1): 58–60.

Major B, Rattazzi L, Brod S, Pilipović I, Leposavić G and D'Acquisto F 2015 Massage-like stroking boosts the immune system in mice. *Sci. Rep.* doi: 10.1038/srep10913.

Marofi M, Sirousfard M, Moeini M and Ghanadi A 2015 Evaluation of the effect of aromatherapy with Rosa damascena Mill. on postoperative pain intensity in hospitalized children in selected hospitals affiliated to Isfahan University of Medical Sciences in 2013: A randomized clinical trial. *Iran. J. Nurs. Midwifery Res. 20*(2): 247–54.

Maruyama N, Ishibashi H, Hu W, Morofuji S *et al.* 2006 Suppression of carrageenan- and collagen II-induced inflammation in mice by geranium oil. *Mediators Inflamm.* doi: 10.1155/MI/2006/62537.

Marzouk TM, El-Nemer AM and Baraka HN 2013 The effect of aromatherapy abdominal massage on alleviating menstrual pain in nursing students: A prospective randomized cross-over study. *Evid. Based Complement. Alternat. Med.* doi: 10.1155/2013/532657.

McGeorge BC and Steele MC 1991 Allergic contact dermatitis of the nipple from Roman chamomile ointment. *Contact Dermatitis 24*(2): 139–40.

McNabb M, Kimber L, Haines A and McCourt C 2006 Does regular massage from late pregnancy to birth decrease maternal pain perception during labour and birth? A feasibility study to investigate a programme of massage, controlled breathing and visualization, from 36 weeks of pregnancy until birth *CTCP 12*(3): 222–31.

Melzack R and Wall PD 1965 Pain mechanisms: A new theory. *Science 150*: 971–9.

Mertas A, Garbusińska A, Szliszka E, Jureczko A, Kowalska M and Król W 2015 The influence of tea tree oil (Melaleuca alternifolia) on fluconazole activity against fluconazole-resistant Candida albicans strains. *Biomed. Res. Int.* doi: 10.1155/2015/590470.

Mertens M, Buettner A and Kirchoff E 2009 The volatile constituents of frankincense – a review. *Flavour and Fragrance Journal 24*: 279–300.

Minaiyan M, Ghannadi A, Asadi M, Etemad M and Mahzouni P 2014 Anti-inflammatory effect of Prunus armeniaca L. (Apricot) extracts ameliorates TNBS-induced ulcerative colitis in rats. *Res. Pharm. Sci. 9*(4): 225–31.

Misharina TA and Polshkov AN 2005 Antioxidant properties of essential oils: Auto-oxidation of essential oils from laurel and fennel and effects of mixing with essential oil from coriander. Article in Russian *Prikladnaia Biokhimia MIkrobiologiia 41*: 693–702, cited by Tisserand and Young 2014 *Essential Oil Safety* (2nd edn): Edinburgh: Churchill Livingstone.

Mitchell DM 2014 Women's use of complementary and alternative medicine in pregnancy: A search for holistic wellbeing *Women Birth 27*(4): 276–80.

Mitchell DM 2015 Women's use of complementary and alternative medicine in pregnancy: Narratives of transformation. *Complement. Ther. Clin. Pract.* doi: 10.1016/j.ctcp.2015.05.006.

Mohebbi Z, Moghadasi M, Homayouni K and Nikou MH 2014 The effect of back massage on blood pressure in the patients with primary hypertension in 2012–2013: A randomized clinical trial. *Int. J. Community Based Nurs. Midwifery* 2(4): 251–8.

Moon HK, Kang P, Lee HS, Min SS and Seol GH 2014 Effects of 1,8-cineole on hypertension induced by chronic exposure to nicotine in rats. *J. Pharm. Pharmacol.* 66(5): 688–93.

Morelli M, Chapman CE and Sullivan SJ 1999 Do cutaneous receptors contribute to the changes in the amplitude of the H-reflex during massage? *Electromyogr. Clin. Neurophysiol.* 39(7): 441–7.

Morhenn V, Beavin LE and Zak PJ 2012 Massage increases oxytocin and reduces adrenocorticotropin hormone in humans. *Altern. Ther. Health Med.* 18(6): 11–18.

Mortazavi SH, Khaki S, Moradi R, Heidari K and Vasegh Rahimparvar SF 2012 Effects of massage therapy and presence of attendant on pain, anxiety and satisfaction during labor. *Arch. Gynecol. Obstet.* 286(1): 19–23.

Moss M, Hewitt S, Moss L and Wesnes K 2008 Modulation of cognitive performance and mood by aromas of peppermint and ylang-ylang. *Int. J. Neurosci.* 118(1): 59–77.

Moss M, Howarth R, Wilkinson L and Wesnes K 2006 Expectancy and the aroma of Roman chamomile influence mood and cognition in healthy volunteers. *International Journal of Aromatherapy* 16: 63–73.

Mostafa DM, Ammar NM, Basha M, Hussein RA, El Awdan S and Awad G 2015 Transdermal microemulsions of Boswellia carterii Bird: Formulation, characterization and in vivo evaluation of anti-inflammatory activity. *Drug Deliv.* 22(6): 748–56.

Muthaiyan A, Biswas D, Crandall PG, Wilkinson BJ and Ricke SC 2012 Application of orange essential oil as an antistaphylococcal agent in a dressing model. *BMC Complement. Altern. Med.* doi: 10.1186/1472-6882-12-125.

Nagai K, Niijima A, Horii Y, Shen J and Tanida M 2014 Olfactory stimulatory with grapefruit and lavender oils change autonomic nerve activity and physiological function. *Auton. Neurosci.* 185: 29–35.

Namazi M, Amir S, Akbari S, Mojab F et al. 2014a Aromatherapy with citrus aurantium oil and anxiety during the first stage of labor. *Iran. Red Crescent Med. J.* 16(6): e18371.

Namazi M, Amir S, Akbari S, Mojab F et al. 2014b Effects of citrus aurantium (bitter orange) on the severity of first-stage labor pain. *Iran. J. Pharm. Res.* 13(3): 1011–18.

National Toxicology Program 2011a Toxicology and carcinogenesis studies of alpha,beta-thujone (CAS No. 76231-76-0) in F344/N rats and B6C3F1 mice (gavage studies). *Natl Toxicol. Program Tech. Rep. Ser.* 570: 1–260.

National Toxicology Program 2011b Toxicology and carcinogenesis studies of pulegone (CAS No. 89-82-7) in F344/N rats and B6C3F1 mice (gavage studies). *Natl Toxicol. Program Tech. Rep. Ser.* 563: 1–201.

Navarra M, Mannucci C, Delbò M and Calapai G 2015 Citrus bergamia essential oil: From basic research to clinical application. *Front. Pharmacol.* doi: 10.3389/fphar.2015.00036.

Nelson NL 2015 Massage therapy: Understanding the mechanisms of action on blood pressure. A scoping review. *J. Am. Soc. Hypertens.* 9(10): 785–93.

NHS Choices 2015a *Complementary and alternative medicine.* Available at www.nhs.uk/Livewell/complementary-alternative-medicine/Pages/complementary-alternative-medicines.aspx, accessed on 14 March 2016.

NHS Choices 2015b *Are complementary therapies safe in pregnancy?* Available at www. nhs.uk/chq/pages/957.aspx, accessed on 14 March 2014.

NHS Institute for Innovation and Improvement 2009 *High impact actions for nursing and midwifery.* Available at www.institute.nhs.uk/building_capability/general/aims/, accessed on 14 March 2016.

NHS Institute for Innovation and Improvement 2013 *Promoting normal birth.* Available at www.institute.nhs.uk/building_capability/general/promoting_normal_birth.html, accessed on 14 March 2016.

NICE (National Institute for Health and Care Excellence) 2014a *Antenatal care* (Clinical Guideline 62) 2008, revised 2014. Available at www.nice.org.uk/guidance/cg62/chapter/1-Guidance, accessed on 7 May 2016.

NICE (National Institute for Health and Care Excellence) 2014b *Intrapartum care: Care of healthy women and their babies during childbirth* (Clinical Guideline 190) Available at www.nice.org.uk/guidance/cg190/evidence/full-guideline-248734765, accessed on 7 May 2016.

Ni CH, Hou WH, Kao CC, Chang ML *et al.* 2013 The anxiolytic effect of aromatherapy on patients awaiting ambulatory surgery: A randomized controlled trial. *Evid. Based Complement. Alternat. Med.* doi: 10.1155/2013/927419.

Ni X, Suhail MM, Yang Q, Cao A *et al.* 2012 Frankincense essential oil prepared from hydrodistillation of Boswellia sacra gum resins induces human pancreatic cancer cell death in cultures and in a xenograft murine model. *BMC Complement. Altern. Med.* doi: 10.1186/1472-6882-12-253.

Nielsen JB 2006 Natural oils affect the human skin integrity and the percutaneous penetration of benzoic acid dose-dependently. *Basic Clin. Pharmacol. Toxicol.* 98(6): 575–81.

Nielsen JB and Nielsen F 2006 Topical use of tea tree oil reduces the dermal absorption of benzoic acid methiocarb. *Arch. Dermatol. Res.* 297: 395–402.

Nisticò S, Ehrlich J, Gliozzi M, Maiuolo J *et al.* 2015 Telomere and telomerase modulation by bergamot polyphenolic fraction in experimental photoageing in human keratinocytes. *J. Biol. Regul. Homeost. Agents* 29(3): 723–8.

Nursing and Midwifery Council (NMC) 2009 *Standards for Pre-registration Midwifery Education.* London: NMC.

Nursing and Midwifery Council (NMC) 2010 *Standards for Administration of Medicines.* London: NMC.

Nursing and Midwifery Council (NMC) 2015 *The Code: Professional Standards of Practice and Behaviour for Nurses and Midwives.* London: NMC.

Oboh G, Ademosun AO, Odubanjo OV and Akinbola IA 2013 Antioxidative properties and inhibition of key enzymes relevant to type-2 diabetes and hypertension by essential oils from black pepper. *Adv. Pharmacol. Sci.* doi: 10.1155/2013/926047.

Oh JY, Park MA and Kim YC 2014 Peppermint oil promotes hair growth without toxic signs. *Toxicol. Res.* 30(4): 297–304.

Olapour A, Behaeen K, Akhondzadeh R, Soltani F, Al Sadat Razavi F and Bekhradi R 2013 The effect of inhalation of aromatherapy blend containing lavender essential oil on Cesarean postoperative pain. *Anesth. Pain Med.* 3(1): 203–7.

Ostad SN, Khakinegad B and Sabzevari O 2004 Evaluation of the teratogenicity of fennel essential oil (FEO) on the rat embryo limb buds culture. *Toxicol. In Vitro 18*(5): 623–7.

Ou MC, Hsu TF, Lai AC, Lin YT and Lin CC 2012 Pain relief assessment by aromatic essential oil massage on outpatients with primary dysmenorrhea: A randomized, double-blind clinical trial. *J. Obstet. Gynaecol. Res. 38*(5): 817–22.

Ou MC, Lee YF, Li CC and Wu SK 2014 The effectiveness of essential oils for patients with neck pain: A randomized controlled study. *J. Altern. Complement. Med. 20*(10): 771–9.

Overman DO and White JA 1983 Comparative teratogenic effects of methyl salicylate applied orally or topically to hamsters. *Teratology 28*(3): 421–6.

Pallivalapila AR, Stewart D, Shetty A, Pande B, Singh R and McLay JS 2015 Use of complementary and alternative medicines during the third trimester. *Obstet. Gynecol. 125*(1): 204–11.

Paulsen E, Chistensen LP and Andersen KE 2008 Cosmetics and herbal remedies with Compositae plant extracts – Are they tolerated by Compositae-allergic patients? *Contact Dermatitis 58*(1): 15–23.

Pazyar N, Yaghoobi R, Bagherani N and Kazerouni A 2013 A review of applications of tea tree oil in dermatology. *Int. J. Dermatol. 52*(7): 784–90.

Peace Rhind J 2012 *Essential Oils: A Handbook for Aromatherapy Practice* (2nd edn). London: Singing Dragon.

Perriam G 2015 Sacred spaces, healing places: Therapeutic landscapes of spiritual significance. *J. Med. Humanit. 36*(1): 19–33.

Perry R, Terry R, Watson LK and Ernst E 2012 Is lavender an anxiolytic drug? A systematic review of randomised clinical trials. *Phytomedicine 19*(8–9): 825–35.

Posadzki P, Alotaibi A and Ernst E 2012 Adverse effects of aromatherapy: A systematic review of case reports and case series. *Int. J. Risk Saf. Med. 24*(3): 147–61.

Raisi Dehkordi Z, Hosseini Baharanchi FS and Bekhradi R 2014 Effect of lavender inhalation on the symptoms of primary dysmenorrhea and the amount of menstrual bleeding: A randomized clinical trial. *Complement. Ther. Med. 22*(2): 212–19.

Ramos Alvarenga RF, Wan B, Inui T, Franzblau SG, Pauli GF and Jaki BU 2014 Airborne antituberculosis activity of Eucalyptus citriodora essential oil. *J. Nat. Prod. 77*(3): 603–10.

Rao RM, Raghuram N, Nagendra HR, Usharani MR *et al.* 2015 Effects of an integrated yoga program on self-reported depression scores in breast cancer patients undergoing conventional treatment: A randomized controlled trial. *Indian J. Palliat. Care 21*(2): 174–81.

Rapaport MH, Schettler P and Bresee C 2012 A preliminary study of the effects of repeated massage on hypothalamic-pituitary-adrenal and immune function in healthy individuals: A study of mechanisms of action and dosage. *J. Altern. Complement. Med. 18*(8): 789–97.

Rashidi Fakari F, Tabatabaeichehr M, Kamali H, Rashidi Fakari F and Naseri M 2015 Effect of inhalation of aroma of geranium essence on anxiety and physiological parameters during first stage of labor in nulliparous women: A randomized clinical trial. *J. Caring Sci. 4*(2): 135–41.

Rath CC, Devi S, Dash SK and Mishra RK 2008 Antibacterial potential assessment of jasmine essential oil against e. Coli. *Indian J. Pharm. Sci. 70*(2): 238–41.

Rehman JU, Ali A and Khan IA 2014 Plant based products: Use and development as repellents against mosquitoes: A review. *Fitoterapia 95*: 65–74.

Roberti di Sarsina P and Tassinari M 2015 Person-centred healthcare and medicine paradigm: It's time to clarify. *EPMA J. 6*(1): 11.

Rudnicki J, Boberski M, Butrymowicz E, Niedbalski P *et al.* 2012 Recording of amplitude-integrated electroencephalography, oxygen saturation, pulse rate, and cerebral blood flow during massage of premature infants. *Am. J. Perinatol. 29*(7): 561–6.

Rutherford T, Nixon R, Tam M and Tate B 2007 Allergy to tea tree oil: Retrospective review of 41 cases with positive patch tests over 4.5 years. *Australas. J. Dermatol. 48*(2): 83–7.

Sadeghi Aval Shahr H, Saadat M, Kheirkhah M and Saadat E 2015 The effect of self-aromatherapy massage of the abdomen on the primary dysmenorrhoea. *J. Obstet. Gynaecol. 35*(4): 382–5.

Saiyudthong S, Ausavarungnirum R, Jiwajinda S and Turakiwanakan W 2009 Effects of aromatherapy massage with lime essential oil on stress. *International Journal of Essential Oil Therapeutics 3*(2): 76–80.

Saiyudthong S and Marsden CA 2011 Acute effects of bergamot oil on anxiety-related behaviour and corticosterone level in rats. *Phytother. Res. 25*(6): 858–62.

Samber N, Khan A, Varma A and Manzoor N 2015 Synergistic anti-candidal activity and mode of action of Mentha piperita essential oil and its major components. *Pharm. Biol. 8*: 1–9.

Santesteban Muruzábal R, Hervella Garcés M, Larrea García M, Loidi Pascual L, Agulló Pérez A and Yanguas Bayona I 2015 Secondary effects of topical application of an essential oil. Allergic contact dermatitis due to tea tree oil. *An. Sist. Sanit. Navar. 38*(1): 163–7.

Sattari M, Dilmaghanizadeh M, Hamishehkar H and Mashayekhi SO 2012 Self-reported use and attitudes regarding herbal medicine safety during pregnancy in Iran. *Jundishapur J. Nat. Pharm. Prod. 7*(2): 45–9.

Satyal P, Shrestha S and Setzer WN 2015 Composition and bioactivities of an (E)-β-farnesene chemotype of chamomile (Matricaria chamomilla) essential oil from Nepal. *Nat. Prod. Commun. 10*(8): 1453–7.

Saunders T 2003 Health hazards and electromagnetic fields. *Complement. Ther. Nurs. Midwifery 9*(4): 191–7.

Sayorwan W, Siripornpanich V, Piriyapunyaporn T, Hongratanaworakit T, Kotchabhakdi N and Ruangrungsi N 2012 The effects of lavender oil inhalation on emotional states, autonomic nervous system, and brain electrical activity. *J. Med. Assoc. Thai. 95*(4): 598–606.

Schaller M and Korting HC 1995 Allergic contact dermatitis from essential oils used in aromatherapy. *Clin. Exp. Dermatol. 20*: 143–5.

Scheinman P 1996 Allergic contact dermatitis to fragrance: A review. *Am J Contact Dermatol 7*: 65–76.

Schneider R 2015 There is something in the air: Testing the efficacy of a new olfactory stress relief method (Aromastick®). *Stress and Health.* doi: 10.1002/smi.2636.

Selim SA, Adam ME, Hassan SM and Albalawi AR 2014 Chemical composition, antimicrobial and antibiofilm activity of the essential oil and methanol extract of the Mediterranean cypress (Cupressus sempervirens L.). *BMC Complement. Altern. Med.* doi: 10.1186/1472-6882-14-179.

Seol GH, Lee YH, Kang P, You JH, Park M and Min SS 2013 Randomized controlled trial for Salvia sclarea or Lavandula angustifolia: Differential effects on blood pressure in female patients with urinary incontinence undergoing urodynamic examination. *J. Altern. Complement. Med.* 19(7): 664–70.

Seol GH, Shim HS, Kim PJ, Moon HK *et al.* 2010 Antidepressant-like effect of Salvia sclarea is explained by modulation of dopamine activities in rats. *J. Ethnopharmacol.* 130(1): 187–90.

Sharpe PA, Wilcox S, Schoffman DE, Hutto B and Ortaglia A 2015 Association of complementary and alternative medicine use with symptoms and physical functional performance among adults with arthritis. *Disabil. Health J.* 9(1): 37–45.

Shavakhi A, Ardestani SK, Taki M, Goli M and Keshteli AH 2012 Premedication with peppermint oil capsules in colonoscopy: A double blind placebo-controlled randomized trial study. *Acta Gastroenterol. Belg.* 75(3): 349–53.

Sheikhan F, Jahdi F, Khoei EM, Shamsalizadeh N, Sheikhan M and Haghani H 2012 Episiotomy pain relief: Use of Lavender oil essence in primiparous Iranian women. *Complement. Ther. Clin. Pract.* 18(1): 66–70.

Shen J, Niijima A, Tanida M, Horii Y, Maeda K and Nagai K 2005 Olfactory stimulation with scent of grapefruit oil affects autonomic nerves, lipolysis and appetite in rats. *Neuroscience Lett.* 380: 289–94.

Sibbritt DW, Catling CJ, Adams J, Shaw AJ and Homer CS 2014 The self-prescribed use of aromatherapy oils by pregnant women. *Women Birth* 27(1): 41–5.

Siddiqui MZ 2011 Boswellia serrata, a potential antiinflammatory agent: An overview. *Indian J. Pharm. Sci.* 73(3): 255–61.

Sienkiewicz M, Głowacka A, Kowalczyk E, Wiktorowska-Owczarek A, Jóźwiak-Bębenista M and Łysakowska M 2014 The biological activities of cinnamon, geranium and lavender essential oils. *Molecules* 19(12): 20929–40.

Silva J, Abebe W, Sousa SM, Duarte VG, Machado MI and Matos FJ 2003 Analgesic and anti-inflammatory effects of essential oils of eucalyptus. *J. Ethnopharmacol.* 89: 277–83.

Sim TF, Sherriff J, Hattingh HL, Parsons R and Tee LB 2013 The use of herbal medicines during breastfeeding: A population-based survey in Western Australia. *BMC Complement. Altern. Med.* doi: 10.1186/1472-6882-13-317.

Smith CA, Collins CT and Crowther CA 2011 Aromatherapy for pain management in labour. *Cochrane Database Syst. Rev.* doi: 10.1002/14651858.CD009215.

Soković M, Glamočlija J, Marin PD, Brkić D and van Griensven LJ 2010 Antibacterial effects of the essential oils of commonly consumed medicinal herbs using an in vitro model. *Molecules* 15(11): 7532–46.

Soltani R, Soheilipour S, Hajhashemi V, Asghari G, Bagheri M and Molavi M 2013 Evaluation of the effect of aromatherapy with lavender essential oil on post-tonsillectomy pain in pediatric patients: A randomized controlled trial. *Int. J. Pediatr. Otorhinolaryngol.* 77(9): 1579–81.

Spadaro F, Costa R, Circosta C and Occhiuto F 2012 Volatile composition and biological activity of key lime Citrus aurantifolia essential oil. *Nat. Prod. Commun.* 7(11): 1523–6.

Spencer KM 2004 The primal touch of birth: Mothers, midwives and massage. *Midwifery Today 70*: 11–14.

Stea S, Beraudi A and De Pasquale D 2014 Essential oils for complementary treatment of surgical patients: State of the art. *Evid. Based Complement. Alternat. Med.* doi: 10.1155/2014/726341.

Stewart D, Pallivalappila AR, Shetty A, Pande B and McLay JS 2014 Healthcare professional views and experiences of complementary and alternative therapies in obstetric practice in North East Scotland: A prospective questionnaire survey. *BJOG 121*(8): 1015–19.

Stringer J and Donald G 2011 Aromasticks in cancer care: An innovation not to be sniffed at. *Complement. Ther. Clin. Pract. 17*(2): 116–21.

Strouss L, Mackley A, Guillen U, Paul DA and Locke R 2014 Complementary and alternative medicine use in women during pregnancy: Do their healthcare providers know? *BMC Complement. Altern. Med.* doi: 10.1186/1472-6882-14-85.

Suhail MM, Wu W, Cao A, Mondalek FG *et al.* 2011 Boswellia sacra essential oil induces tumor cell-specific apoptosis and suppresses tumor aggressiveness in cultured human breast cancer cells. *BMC Complement. Altern. Med.* doi: 10.1186/1472-6882-11-129.

Tadtong S, Kamkaen N, Watthanachaiyingcharoen R and Ruangrungsi N 2015 Chemical components of four essential oils in aromatherapy recipe. *Nat. Prod. Commun. 10*(6): 1091–2.

Takahashi M, Yamanaka A, Asanuma C, Asano H, Satou T and Koike K 2014 Anxiolytic-like effect of inhalation of essential oil from Lavandula officinalis: Investigation of changes in 5-HT turnover and involvement of olfactory stimulation. *Nat. Prod. Commun. 9*(7): 1023–6.

Tan LT, Lee LH, Yin WF, Chan CK *et al.* 2015 Traditional uses, phytochemistry, and bioactivities of Cananga odorata (ylang-ylang). *Evid. Based Complement. Alternat. Med.* doi: 10.1155/2015/896314.

Tanida M, Niijima A, Shen J, Nakamura T and Nagai K 2006 Olfactory stimulation with scent of lavender oil affects autonomic neurotransmission and blood pressure in rats. *Neurosci Lett. 398*(1–2): 155–60.

Tee BC, Chortos A, Berndt A, Nguyen AK *et al.* 2015 A skin-inspired organic digital mechanoreceptor. *Science 350*(6258): 313–16.

Tester-Dalderup CBM 1980 Drugs Used in Bronchial Asthma and Cough. In Dukes (ed.) *Meyler's Side Effects of Drugs* (9th edition) Amsterdam: Excerpta Medica.

Thomas I (ed.) 1993 *Culpeper's Book of Birth*. London: Grange Publishing.

Thompson A, Meah D, Ahmed N, Conniff-Jenkins R *et al.* 2013 Comparison of the antibacterial activity of essential oils and extracts of medicinal and culinary herbs to investigate potential new treatments for irritable bowel syndrome. *BMC Complement. Altern. Med.* doi: 10.1186/1472-6882-13-338.

Tiran D 2004 Viewpoint–midwives' enthusiasm for complementary therapies: A cause for concern? *Complement. Ther. Nurs. Midwifery 10*(2): 77–9.

Tiran D 2010a Complementary therapies and the NMC. *Pract. Midwife 13*(5): 4–5.

Tiran D 2010b *Reflexology in Pregnancy and Childbirth*. Edinburgh: Elsevier Science.

Tiran D 2011a The need to include the subject of natural remedies in midwifery education. *Complement. Ther. Clin. Pract. 17*(4): 187–8.

Tiran D 2011b Smell's good! *Practising Midwife 14*(10): 11–15.

Tiran D 2012 Ginger to reduce nausea and vomiting during pregnancy: Evidence of effectiveness is not the same as proof of safety. *Complement. Ther. Clin. Pract. 18*(1): 22–5.

Tiran D 2014 *Aromatherapy in Midwifery Practice: A Manual for Clinical Practice.* London: Expectancy.

Tisserand R (ed.) 1993 *Gattefosse's Aromatherapy: The First Book on Aromatherapy* (translated from the French). Saffron Walden: CW Daniel.

Tisserand R and Young R 2014 *Essential Oil Safety* (2nd edn). Edinburgh: Churchill Livingstone.

Tomić M, Popović V, Petrović S, Stepanović-Petrović R *et al.* 2014 Antihyperalgesic and antiedematous activities of bisabolol-oxides-rich matricaria oil in a rat model of inflammation. *Phytother. Res. 28*(5): 759–66.

Törnhage CJ, Skogar Ö, Borg A, Larsson B *et al.* 2013 Short- and long-term effects of tactile massage on salivary cortisol concentrations in Parkinson's disease: A randomised controlled pilot study. *BMC Complement. Altern. Med.* doi: 10.1186/1472-6882-13-357.

Trabace L, Tucci P, Ciuffreda L, Matteo M *et al.* 2015 'Natural' relief of pregnancy-related symptoms and neonatal outcomes: Above all do no harm. *J. Ethnopharmacol. 174*: 396–402.

Umezu T 2012 Evaluation of the effects of plant-derived essential oils on central nervous system function using discrete shuttle-type conditioned avoidance response in mice. *Phytother. Res. 26*(6): 884–91.

Uvnäs-Moberg K 2011 *The Oxytocin Factor*. London: Pinter and Martin.

Vakilian K, Atarha M, Bekhradi R and Chaman R 2011 Healing advantages of lavender essential oil during episiotomy recovery: A clinical trial. *Complement. Ther. Clin. Pract. 17*(1): 50–3.

Valnet J 1980 *The Practice of Aromatherapy: A Classic Compendium of Plant Medicines and Their Healing Properties* (ed. R Tisserand). Saffron Walden: CW Daniel.

Varney E and Buckle J 2013 Effect of inhaled essential oils on mental exhaustion and moderate burnout: A small pilot study. *J. Altern. Complement. Med. 19*(1): 69–71.

Warnke PH, Lott AJ, Sherry E, Wiltfang J and Podschun R 2013 The ongoing battle against multi-resistant strains: In-vitro inhibition of hospital-acquired MRSA, VRE, Pseudomonas, ESBL E. coli and Klebsiella species in the presence of plant-derived antiseptic oils. *J. Craniomaxillofac. Surg. 41*(4): 321–6.

Warriner S, Bryan K and Brown AM 2014 Women's attitude towards the use of complementary and alternative medicines (CAM) in pregnancy. *Midwifery 30*(1): 138–43.

Watanabe E, Kuchta K, Kimura M, Rauwald HW, Kamei T and Imanishi J 2015 Effects of bergamot (Citrus bergamia (Risso) Wright & Arn.) essential oil aromatherapy on mood states, parasympathetic nervous system activity, and salivary cortisol levels in 41 healthy females. *Forsch. Komplementmed. 22*(1): 43–9.

Woollard AC, Tatham KC and Barker S 2007 The influence of essential oils on the process of wound healing: A review of the current evidence. *J. Wound Care 16*(6): 255–7.

Wu JJ, Cui Y, Yang YS, Kang MS *et al.* 2014 Modulatory effects of aromatherapy massage intervention on electroencephalogram, psychological assessments, salivary cortisol and plasma brain-derived neurotrophic factor. *Complement. Ther. Med.* 22(3): 456–62.

Wyllie JP and Alexander FW 1994 Nasal instillation of Olbas oil in an infant. *Arch. Dis. Childhood* 70: 357–8.

Yang HJ, Kim KY, Kang P, Lee HS and Seol GH 2014 Effects of Salvia sclarea on chronic immobilization stress induced endothelial dysfunction in rats. *BMC Complement. Altern. Med.* doi: 10.1186/1472-6882-14-396.

Yates S 2003 *Shiatsu for Midwives.* Edinburgh: Churchill Livingstone.

Yates S 2010 *Pregnancy and Childbirth: An Holistic Approach to Massage and Bodywork.* Edinburgh: Churchill Livingstone.

Yavari Kia P, Safajou F, Shahnazi M and Nazemiyeh H 2014 The effect of lemon inhalation aromatherapy on nausea and vomiting of pregnancy: A double-blinded, randomized, controlled clinical trial. *Iran. Red Crescent Med. J.* doi: 10.5812/ircmj.14360.

Yemele MD, Telefo PB, Lienou LL, Tagne SR *et al.* 2015 Ethnobotanical survey of medicinal plants used for pregnant women's health conditions in Menoua division-West Cameroon. *J. Ethnopharmacol.* 160: 14–31.

Yosipovitch G, Xiong GI, Haus E, Sackett-Lundeen L, Ashkenazi I and Maibach HI 1998 Time dependent variations of the skin barrier function in humans: Trans-epidermal water loss, stratum corneum hydration, skin surface pH and skin temperature. *J. Invest. Dermatol.* 110: 22–3.

Zabirunnisa M, Gadagi JS, Gadde P, Myla N, Koneru J and Thatimatla C 2014 Dental patient anxiety: Possible deal with Lavender fragrance. *J. Res. Pharm. Pract.* 3(3): 100–3.

Zargaran A, Borhani-Haghighi A, Faridi P, Daneshamouz S, Kordafshari G and Mohagheghzadeh A 2014 Potential effect and mechanism of action of topical chamomile (Matricaria chammomila L.) oil on migraine headache: A medical hypothesis. *Med Hypotheses* 83(5): 566–9.

Subject Index

Author Index